:ching and
ngthening Exercises

Stretching and Strengthening Exercises

Hans Spring, Urs Illi, Hans-Ruedi Kunz
Karl Röthlin, Werner Schneider
and Thomas Tritschler

105 illustrations

1991
Georg Thieme Verlag Stuttgart · New York
Thieme Medical Publishers, Inc., New York

Hans Spring, M.D.,
Medical Director
Clinic for Rheumatology and
  Rehabilitation
3954 Leukerbad, Switzerland

Urs Illi
Swiss Association for
  Sport in Schools
ETH Center
8092 Zurich, Switzerland

Hans-Ruedi Kunz
Biomechanics Laboratory
ETH Center
8092 Zurich, Switzerland

Karl Röthlin
Physiotherapist
Flurstrasse 15
8048 Zurich, Switzerland

Werner Schneider, M.D.
Hauptstrasse 39
8280 Kreuzlingen, Switzerland

Thomas Tritschler
Director
Physiotherapy School
Kantonsspital
8208 Schaffhausen, Switzerland

Translator:
Gerhard S. Sharon
4525 Henry Hudson Parkway
Riverdale, N.Y. 10471, USA

Illustrations:
Gabriela Kupferschmidt

Cover design by
Dominique Loenicker

© 1991 Georg Thieme Verlag
Rüdigerstrasse 14,
D-70469 Stuttgart, Germany
Thieme Medical Publishers, Inc.,
381 Park Avenue South, New York,
N.Y. 10016

Typeset and printed in Germany by
Druckhaus Götz GmbH,
D-71636 Ludwigsburg

ISBN 3-13-753301-5 (GTV, Stuttgart)
ISBN 0-86577-366-1 (TMP, New York)
          2   3   4   5   6

Library of Congress Cataloging-in-Publication Data

Dehn- und Kräftigungsgymnastik. English.
  Stretching and strengthening exercises / Hans Spring
  … [et al.] ;
      p.   cm.
  Translation of: Dehn- und Kräftigungsgymnastik.
  Includes bibliographical references.
  Includes index.
  ISBN 3-13-753301-5. – – ISBN 0-86577-366-1
  1. Stretching exercises.   I. Spring, Hans.   II. Title.
  [DNLM: 1. Exercise. 2. Muscles. 3. Sports Medicine.
  WE 500
D322s]
RA781.63.D4413   1991
613.7'1–dc20
DNLM/DLC   90–11260
for Library of Congress   CIP

Important Note: Medicine is an ever-changing science. Research and clinical experience are continually broadening our knowledge, in particular our knowledge of proper treatment and drug therapy. Insofar as this book mentions any dosage or application, readers may rest assured that the authors, editors and publishers have made every effort to ensure that such references are strictly in accordance with the **state of knowledge at the time of production of the book. Nevertheless, every user is requested** to examine carefully the manufacturer's leaflets accompanying each drug to check on his own responsibility whether the dosage schedules recommended therein or the contraindications stated by the manufacturers differ from the statements made in the present book. Such examination is particularly important with drugs that are either rarely used or have been newly released on the market.

This book is an authorized and revised translation from the 2nd German edition, published and copyrighted 1988 by Georg Thieme Verlag, Stuttgart, Germany. Title of the German edition: Dehn- und Kräftigungsgymnastik. Stretching und dynamische Kräftigung.

Preface

Stretching exercises have taken on considerable importance in sports and rehabilitation in recent years.

A wide variety of underlying theoretical and practical principles are discussed in the literature. The concept presented here includes theoretical principles as well as practical instructions for performing these stretching and strengthening exercises. It addresses athletes as well as trainers, physical education specialists, physical therapists, and physicians caring for athletes.

The team of authors consists of two physicians and two physical therapists, all active in sports medicine and manual medicine, one decathlon trainer with a doctorate in biomechanics, and a teacher of physical education instructors. We are therefore well equipped to answer questions on this topic competently and comprehensively.

Important new aspects of stretching and strengthening exercises in sports are presented by introducing the concepts of "muscular imbalance" and "neuromuscular stretching techniques." Scientific and neurophysiologic factors are duly taken into account in these exercises. They are designed to achieve and maintain muscular balance so as to minimize susceptibility to injury and the occurrence of sports injuries, and to enhance performance capabilities.

The first, practical part describes the basic rules to be observed to execute the stretching and strenghtening exercises properly. The second part deals with the theoretical background for muscle stretching and strengthening.

We should like to take this opportunity to thank our artist, Mrs. G. Kupferschmidt, for her valued collaboration; it is, in fact, the up-to-date, easily comprehensible illustrations which make this exercise book come alive. We are grateful for the assistance given us by the Thieme Verlag, and in particular by Mr. A. Menge and his associates.

Leukerbad, in August 1990   *H. Spring, U. Illi, H.-R. Kunz,*
                                K. Röthlin, W. Schneider,
                                T. Tritschler

Contents

Introduction

Every physical performance is made up of one or more of the basic constitutional factors of strength, endurance, mobility, speed and coordination. The greater the complexity of the sports activity or discipline, the greater the number of constitutional factors that are involved and can have a restrictive effect on performance (Fig. 1).

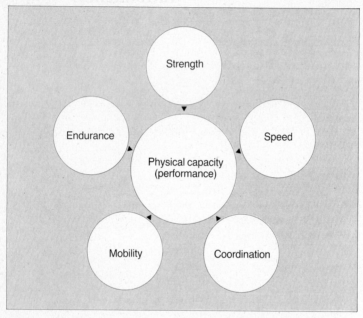

Fig. 1   Constitutional factors underlying physical peformance

Of course, other factors, such as body habitus, mental characteristics, and technical and tactical skills, all critically influence one's overall athletic performance. However, we are not concerned with these aspects here.

Each constitutional factor can be trained selectively. How much weight is attached to individual factors in training depends on the requirements, as determined by the specific sports activity.

Athletes aiming for fitness can confine their efforts to promoting endurance, strength and mobility, and with appropriate training will improve their overall physical performance (Fig. 2).

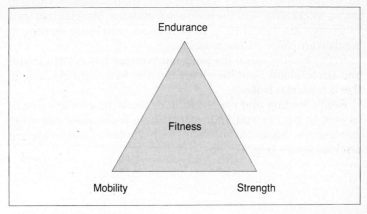

Fig. 2   Constitutional factors needed to achieve a high degree of fitness

Even athletes who have set their sights higher, regardless of the type of sports activity, can never dispense with a basic training in endurance, strength and mobility.

It is the purpose of this book to help improve two of these properties, namely, mobility and strength.

Specific muscle groups have been identified and selected since experience has shown that certain muscle groups are frequently "forgotten", or are at least trained incorrectly, in the usual flexibility and strength training. It is precisely these "forgotten" and incorrectly trained muscles that can lead to musculoskeletal complaints or cause diminished performance.

If flexibility and strength training is carried out inadequately or incorrectly, this will show itself in two ways: muscles can either become shortened or weakened.

On the one hand, it is necessary to identify and make a distinction between muscles that show reduced length or stretching ability — that is, those that have shortened — and on the other hand, muscles that have reduced strength — those that have weakened.

Apart from developmental or congenital factors, the nerve supply of muscles varies with the different reactions — shortening or weakening — of the individual muscles. Muscles that tend to shorten are described as *tonic muscles,* and those tending to weaken are called *phasic muscles.*

In the healthy state, the tonic musculature has normal length and stretchability, and the phasic muscles have normal strength: this is muscular balance.

Faulty loading and overexertion of the locomotor apparatus, as well as injuries and improper training techniques, can upset this balance. *Muscular imbalance* with shortened and weakened muscles results (Fig. 3).

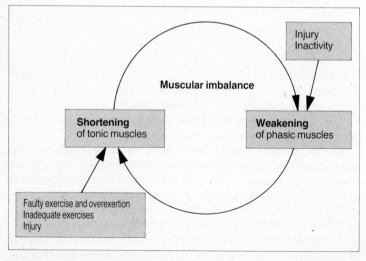

Fig. 3   Muscular imbalance

This muscular imbalance represents a typical vicious circle: The shortening aggravates the weakening, and conversely the weakening aggravates the shortening. When the condition has progressed, the precipitating factor can later in many cases no longer be identified.

Athletes frequently exhibit a muscular imbalance of this sort. The principal causes are one-sided, improper exertion and over-exertion and, not uncommonly, inadequate exercises.

Muscular imbalance reduces the exercise tolerance of the locomotor apparatus. Muscular susceptibility to injury increases: there is a growing incidence of muscle strain and symptoms involving tendon insertions. The joints and spine are overloaded as a result of the disturbed muscular interplay, and states of irritation develop. Muscular imbalance adversely affects performance.

Muscular imbalance, with all its adverse effects, can be remedied or prevented by specific stretching and strengthening exercises (Fig. 4). The stretching and strengthening exercises presented in this book have been chosen with this purpose in mind.

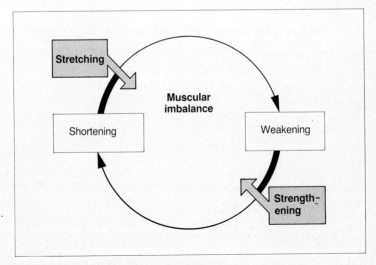

Fig. 4   Influencing muscular imbalance

7

*Directions
for Stretching and
Strengthening
Exercises*

The stretching and strengthening exercises are divided into two sections:

1. Basic program ("Top Ten").
2. Systematic exercise program.

The theoretical part at the end of the book is designed to help you understand the exercises better, but is not necessary to perform them successfully.

Basic Program ("Top Ten")

The basic program comprises 10 stretching exercises targeting the most important muscle groups. The exercises have been chosen so that they can be carried out anywhere in a standing position without any additional equipment. This minimum program allows selective stretching exercises for the most important muscles to be carried out in a short time.

If problems should arise with any muscle group in the course of this basic program, additional exercises from the systematic exercise program should be selected. Individual exercises can also be replaced by ones from the systematic program. Normal stretching capacity can be achieved only if the muscle group in question is stretched in a variety of exercises and with sufficient intensity.

Strengthening exercises should supplement the basic program. These are chosen according to criteria specific to each particular type of sports activity. Selective strengthening of the trunk musculature is necessary in all cases.

Objective of Top Ten Exercises
Maintaining muscular balance.

Systematic Exercise Program

This program is called systematic because it includes stretching and strengthening exercises for every muscle group. The anatomy and function of the principal muscles are described in more detail in this section for better comprehension. Additional information is provided about medical and functional aspects and specific types of sports.

The strengthening exercises shown are meant to be done with a partner. Many of them, however, can be done in the same way, or in a modified form, without a partner. The chosen method of training for strength ist the dynamic slow method.

The stretching exercises can be carried out by three techniques: *Passive static stretching, active static stretching,* and the contract–relax–stretch method. For daily exercises, the passive static form is sufficient to maintain normal muscle length. When there is muscular imbalance, including the contract–relax–stretch maneuver and active static stretching in the exercise program is advantageous. The guiding principle to be observed is: stretching comes before strengthening.

Objective of Systematic Exercise Program

Individualized formulation of a selective exercise program to achieve and maintain muscular balance.

How to Stretch

Passive Static Stretching

Assume the stretch position shown.

Slowly change position in the direction of the arrows, thus increasing the stretch.

Avoid abrupt movements (no bouncing!)

A mild tugging sensation in the muscle being stretched is normal.

Maintain this position for 15–30 seconds.

Breathe calmly and regularly.

Try to relax.

Contract−Relax−Stretch

Assume the stretch position shown.

Tighten (contract) the muscle for 3−7 seconds against resistance (isometric muscle tension).

Then relax the muscle and stretch it further for 10 seconds.

Starting from this new stretched position, carry out isometric contraction and stretching again.

This procedure is repeated 2−3 times.

Active Static Stretching

Assume the stretch position shown.

Slowly tighten the antagonist, thus actively increasing the stretch.

Avoid jerky movements.

A mild tugging sensation in the muscle being stretched is normal.

Maintain the newly reached position for 10−20 seconds.

Breathe calmly and regularly.

Try to relax.

How to Strengthen

Dynamic Slow Training for Strength

Assume the starting position shown. Gradually overcome your partner's resistance by contracting the muscle at a slow but constant rate of movement.

At the end of the contraction, change the direction of motion. You are now blocking your partner's counterforce. At the end of the counteraction, resume contracting the muscle so as to overcome the force exerted by your partner.

Repeat this cycle 10 times.

Perform 2–3 sets of these cycles with rest periods in between.

When to Stretch

Stretch regularly! Only properly and frequently performed stretching exercises will have the desired effect.

Stretch on the following occasions:

— Daily exercises (aerobics, etc.)
— Running, warm-up
— Running, warm-down
— Recovery phase after severe physical stress (the day after)
— Flexibility training.

Watch your body's reaction to the stretching exercises. With time, you will find out what the best time to do the stretching exercises is for you personally — depending on your constitution, state of training, and the type of sports you engage in.

When to Strengthen

The strengthening exercises presented here supplement the stretching exercises. They thus bring about an optimal, well-balanced performance of your muscles and so prevent muscular imbalance from developing. Selected strengthening exercises should be part of your daily exercises. You may, of course, supplement these strengthening exercises at any time with other exercises that are specific for the sports discipline you are active in.

Basic Program "Top Ten"

10 stretching exercises
for the most important
muscle groups.
These can be performed
anywhere and without
any aids.

Top Ten 1

Calf Muscles

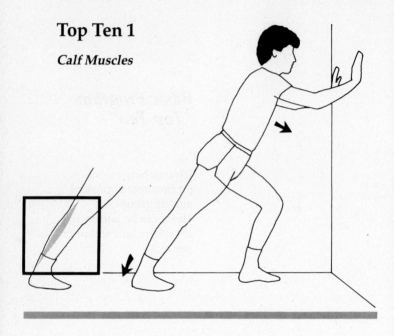

✔ Press your heel against the ground

↘ Lean your body evenly forward

See also pages 30–34 in the systematic exercise program

Top Ten 2

Anterior
Thigh Muscles

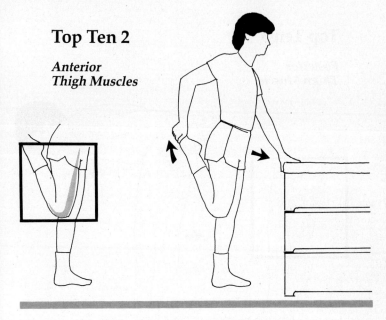

↑ Pull your foot towards your buttocks

↘ Move your pelvis forward

See also pages 35–42 in the systematic exercise program

Top Ten 3

Posterior
Thigh Muscle

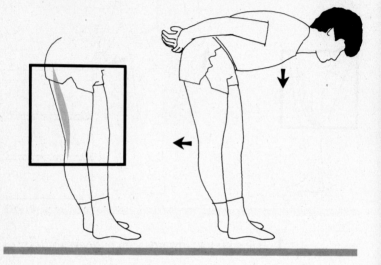

← Stretch your knees

↓ Bend forward at the waist

See also pages 43–49 in the systematic exercise program

Top Ten 4

Anterior
Hip Muscles

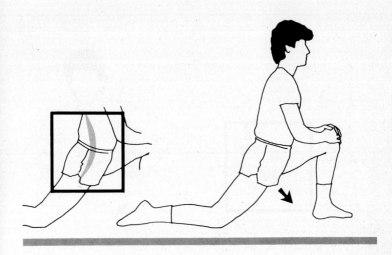

➘ Move your hip forward and downward

See also pages 50–55 in the systematic exercise program

Top Ten 5

Medial Hip Muscles

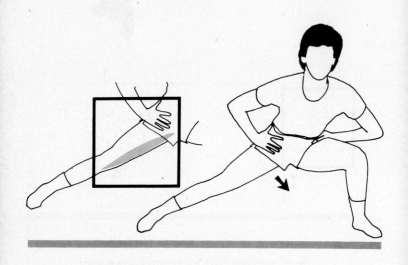

↘ Move your pelvis obliquely downward

See also pages 56–60 in the systematic exercise program

Top Ten 6

Posterior
Hip Muscles

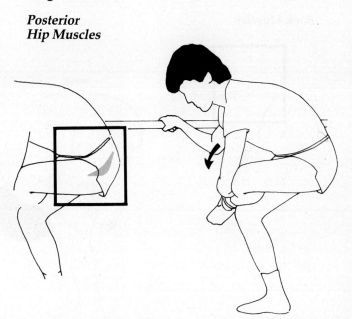

← Bend your trunk forward at the waist

See also pages 61–71 in the systematic exercise program

Top Ten 7

Back Muscles

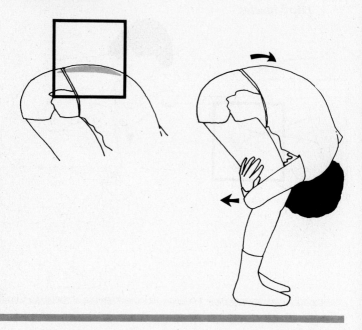

← Stretch your knees

↪ *Bend your back forward*

See also pages 72–76 in the systematic exercise program

Top Ten 8

*Lateral Trunk
Muscles*

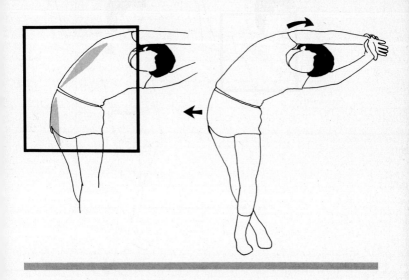

← Move your hip sideways

⤳ Pull your trunk toward the opposite side

See also pages 81–84 in the systematic exercise program

Top Ten 9

Chest Muscles

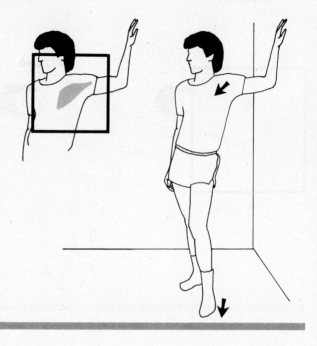

🡧 Take a step forward with the leg on the same side

🡧 Move your shoulder forward

See also pages 85–88 in the systematic exercise program

Top Ten 10

Shoulder Girdle Muscles

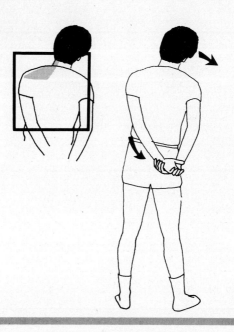

↘ Bend head toward the opposite side

↘ Pull your arm downward

See also pages 89–93 in the systematic exercise program

Systematic Exercise Program

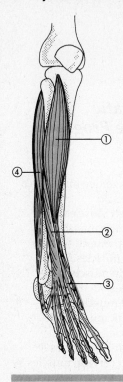

Anterior Leg Muscles (Dorsiflexors)

① Anterior tibialis muscle

② Long extensor muscle of the toes (extensor digitorum longus muscle)

③ Long extensor muscle of the great toe (extensor hallucis longus muscle)

④ Long and short peroneal muscle (peroneus longus and brevis muscles)

Function   — Dorsiflexion (raising) of the foot

①②③   — Inversion of the foot
                (raising the medial margin of the foot)

Function   — Eversion of the foot
                (raising the lateral margin of the foot)

            — Plantar flexion (lowering) of the foot

Notes   — The anterior tibialis muscle, together with the long peroneal muscle, forms a stirrup-like loop which supports the transverse arch of the foot.

            — During sports activities, the foot is subjected to considerable stress. Its normal functioning — locomotion and shock absorption — is assured only as long as the musculature stabilizing the foot has sufficient strength. This explains the importance of regular foot exercises!

            — Specific strengthening of the peroneal muscles is necessary, particularly if there is a tendency for frequent spraining of the ankle joints to occur due to exaggerated outward movement of the foot ("inversion trauma").

Anterior Lower Leg Muscles

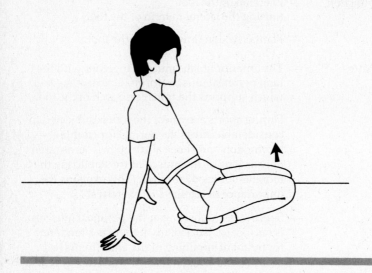

Technique	Passive static stretch
Execution	↖ Raise knees slightly
Notes	— In this exercise, the anterior joint capsule of the ankle joint is quickly placed under tensile stress. The stretching should therefore not be overdone.
	— The anterior leg muscles are also stretched in the stretching exercise on p. 37 (anterior thigh musculature).

*Anterior
Lower Leg Muscles*

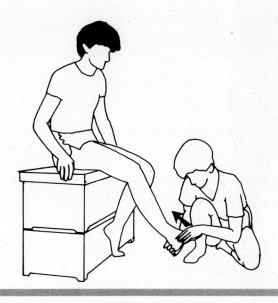

Technique	Dynamic slow strengthening
Execution	↖ Raise your foot
Note	— Raising the lateral margin of the foot with the toes flexed specifically strengthens the peroneal muscles (calf muscles). This strengthening exercise is especially important to avert sprains and strains at the ankle joint.

Calf Muscles

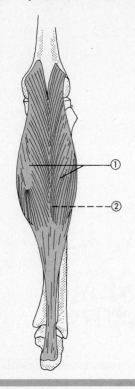

① Gastrocnemius muscle

② Soleus muscle (concealed)

Function — Plantar flexion (lowering) of the foot

— Inversion of the foot (raising the medial margin of the foot)

— Knee flexion (gastrocnemius muscle)

Notes

— Together, the gastrocnemius muscle and the soleus muscle beneath it are called the triceps surae muscle.

— The triceps surae muscle is a tonic (as opposed to phasic) muscle, and tends to shorten.

— The gastrocnemius muscle is a biarticular muscle. The best stretching is done with the knee extended.

— The soleus muscle is a uniarticular muscle. It can be selectively stretched with the knee in flexion.

— The triceps surae muscle is the strongest inverter of the foot (raising the medial foot margin). When it is shortened, the risk of an exaggerated outward movement of the foot ("inversion trauma") is increased.

— Tretment for a painful Achilles tendon (achillodynia) should include stretching exercises for the triceps surae muscle.

Calf Muscles

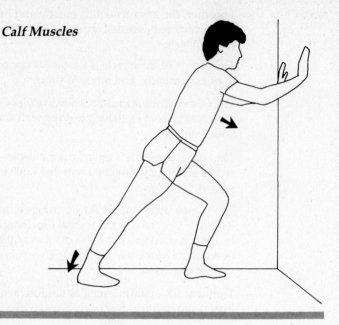

Technique	Passive static stretching
Execution	← Press your heel down on the floor
	↑ Lean your body evenly forward
Note	— If the knee joint is bent in the same exercise, the deep calf muscle (soleus muscle) is stretched selectively.

Calf Muscles

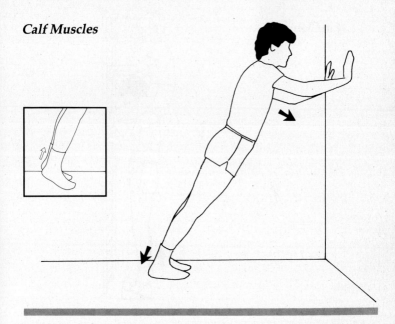

Technique	Contract–relax–stretch
Execution	Stand on toes (3–7 seconds of isometric contraction)
	Relax
	Press the heels down on the floor
	Bend elbows and lean the body forward (stretch for 10 seconds)
	Repeat 2–3 times
Note	— When the knees are flexed, the deep calf muscles (soleus muscles) in particular are stretched.

Calf Muscles

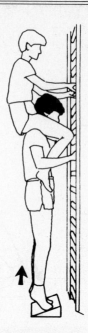

Technique	Dynamic slow strengthening
Execution	↑ Stand on toes
Notes	— Standing on a slanting surface allows a wider range of motion in the ankle joint.
	— The knees remain extended.
	— To increase the load, the exercise may be done one leg at a time.

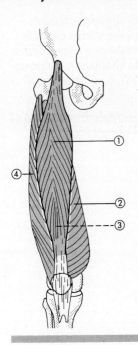

Anterior Thigh Muscles

① Rectus femoris muscle

② Vastus medialis muscle

③ Vastus intermedius muscle (concealed)

④ Vastus lateralis muscle

Function
— Extension of the knee

— Flexion of the hip (rectus femoris muscle)

Notes
— The rectus femoris and the vastus medialis, intermedius, and lateralis muscles form the quadriceps muscle of the thigh (four-headed extensor of the thigh).

— The rectus femoris muscle is a biarticular muscle. It is a tonic muscle, and tends to shorten.

— The vastus medialis muscle is decidedly phasic, and very often reacts by weakening, especially in knee injuries.

— Concurrent shortening of the recuts femoris muscle and weakening of the vastus medialis muscle may be either a cause or a consequence of abnormal cartilaginous changes at the posterior surface of the patella (i. e., patellar chondropathy).

— Treatment for patellar disorders should include selective stretching and strengthening exercises.

Anterior Thigh Muscles

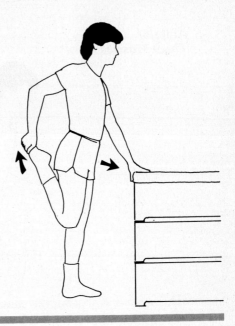

Technique	Passive static stretching
Execution	↑ Pull the foot toward the buttocks
	→ Move the pelvis forward
Notes	— Holding the forefoot stretches the anterior leg muscles as well.
	— Leaning backward excessively as the pelvis moves forward should be avoided.

Anterior Thigh Muscles

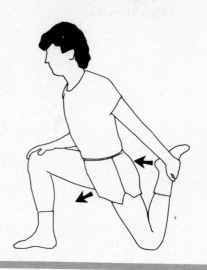

Technique	Passive static stretching
Execution	↙ Move the hip forward
	← Pull the heel toward the buttocks
Notes	— To ensure stability, the free hand may be placed on the floor to give support.
	— Soft padding under the resting knee may prevent unpleasant pressure pain.

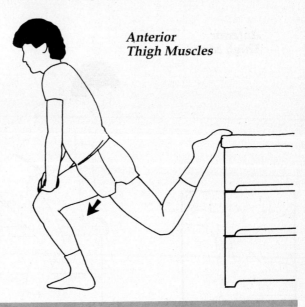

*Anterior
Thigh Muscles*

Technique	Passive static stretch
Execution	🡖 Flex the knee of the upright leg and move the hip forward and downward
Note	— In this exercise, the rectus femoris muscle is stretched by using the hip joint instead of the knee joint.
	This relieves pressure on the knee joint, so that this exercise can also be carried out by those with knee disorders.

Anterior Thigh Muscles

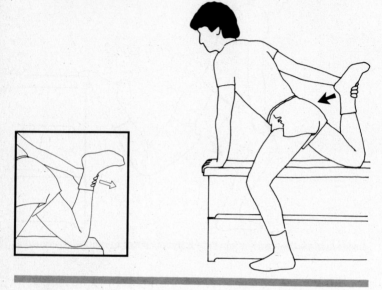

Technique	Contract–relax–stretch
Execution	⟿ Push the lower leg backward against the hand grasping it (3–7 seconds of isometric contraction)
	Relax
	← Pull the heel toward the buttocks (stretch for 10 seconds)
	Repeat 2–3 times
Note	— This position provides good stabilization of the body, so that evasive movements are prevented.

*Anterior
Thigh Muscles*

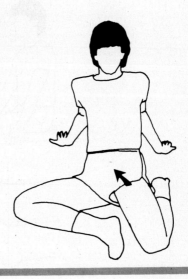

Technique	Active static stretch
Execution	↖ Actively stretch the hip forward and upward
Note	— The back should remain straight. Avoid bending the small of the back too much.

Anterior Thigh Muscles

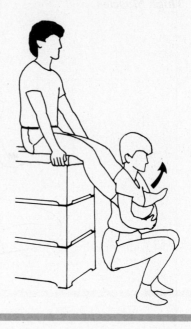

Technique	Dynamic slow strengthening
Execution	↗ Extend the knee
Notes	— The joint should by moved through its entire range of motion.
	— Your partner can reduce the load by actively stretching the knees, or increase it by pushing the feet forward.

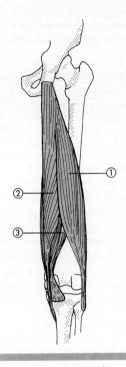

Posterior Thigh Muscles

① Biceps muscle of the thigh (biceps femoris)

② Semitendinous muscle

③ Semimembranous muscle

Function

— Flexion of the knee

— Extension of the hip

— Rotation of the lower leg with the knee flexed (external rotation: biceps femoris; internal rotation: semitendinous and semimembranous muscles)

Notes

— The biceps femoris muscle and the semitendinous and semimembranous muscles are also known as the hamstrings or ischiocrural musculature.

— The hamstring muscles react tonically and tend to shorten.

— Shortening of these muscles often causes muscle strains.

— The way the thigh muscles are usually exercised causes the knee extensors (the quadriceps muscles of the thigh) to be strengthened more intensively than the knee flexors (hamstring muscles). This disproportion between the strength of the extensors and the flexors can lead to an increased susceptibility to injury. Therefore, specific strengthening exercises are needed for the flexors. When measured dynamometrically with the CYBEX machine, the normal flexor force is 60–70% of the extensor force.

Posterior
Thigh Muscles

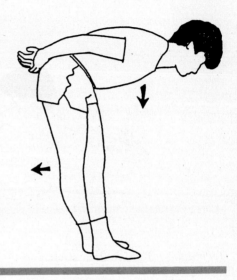

Technique	Passive static stretching
Execution	← Stretch the knee
	↓ Lean forward from the waist
Notes	— Keep the back as straight as possible.
	— Differences in tension between the left and the right side should tell you which side needs to be stretched more intensively.

Posterior Thigh Muscles

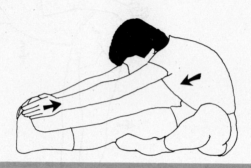

Technique	Passive static stretching
Execution	✔ With the leg straight, tilt your pelvis and trunk forward
Note	— Simultaneously pulling on the foot (→) will stretch the calf musculature.

*Posterior
Thigh Muscles*

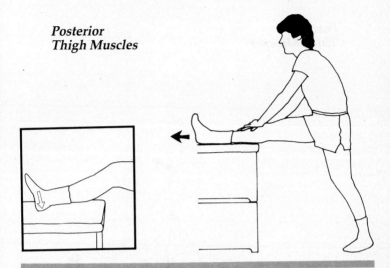

Technique	Contract–relax–stretch
Execution	With the knee slightly bent, press your heel down against the support (3–7 seconds of isometric contraction)
	Relax
	← Straighten the knee and hold it down with the hands. Move your leg forward (away from you) on the support (stretch for 10 seconds)
	Repeat 2–3 times
Note	— To intensify the stretching, increase hip flexion by leaning forward with the trunk.

Posterior Thigh Muscles

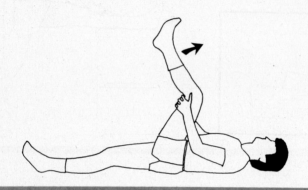

Technique	Active static stretch
Execution	↗ Actively extend the knee with the thigh held in hip flexion
Note	— Flexion of the hip is not altered during the stretch.

*Posterior
Thigh Muscles*

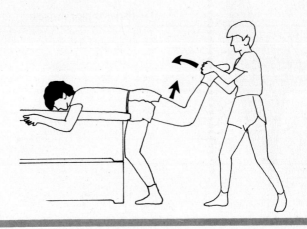

Technique	Dynamic slow strengthening
Execution	↑ Extend the hip actively; the thigh is then held in this position
	↖ Bend the knee
Notes	— This exercise allows isolated strengthening of the posterior thigh musculature. Active extension of the hip bypasses the hip flexor muscles. An arched back should be avoided.
	— At the same time, the hip extensors (gluteus maximus and gluteus medius muscles) are statically strengthened.

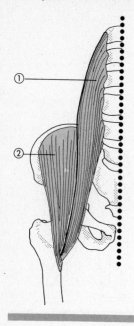

Anterior Hip Muscles

① Psoas major muscle

② Iliac muscle

Function
① + ②

— Flexion of the hip

Function
①

— Stabilization of the lumbar spine

Notes
— Together, these two muscles have become known as the iliopsoas muscle.
The psoas major muscle arises at the lower thoracic and lumbar spine, while the iliac muscle originates on the medial side of the wing of the iliac bone.

— The iliopsoas muscle is the main hip flexor. When the thigh is extended, it tilts the pelvis forward.

— The psoas major muscle has the important function of stabilizing the lumbar spine when the back extensors in the lumbar spine contract at the same time.

— The iliopsoas muscle reacts in a decidedly tonic fashion and tends to shorten, often causing low back pain. Back pain is more severe when the hip extensors (the gluteus medius and gluteus maximus muscles) are weak.

Anterior
Hip Muscles

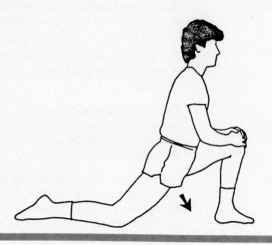

Technique	Passive static stretching
Execution	↘ Press the hip forward and down
Notes	— The feet should remain straight (parallel, forward and backward). Rotation of the hip as an evasive maneuver should be avoided.
	— One may also lean the trunk further forward.

*Anterior
Hip Muscles*

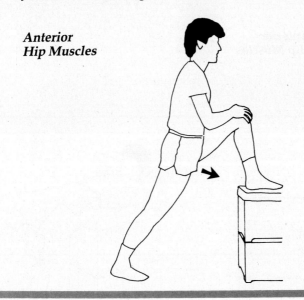

Technique   Passive static stretching

Execution   ➘ Push hip forward

Note   — For selective stretching of the hip flexors only,
              the hip must not be externally rotated. The feet
              continue to point straight forward.

Anterior
Hip Muscles

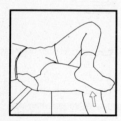

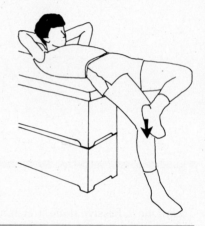

Technique	Contract–relax–stretch
Execution	⇧ Press the freely hanging thigh upward against the resistance of the crossed-over foot (3–7 seconds of isometric contraction)
	Relax
	⬇ Press down onto the thigh with the foot (stretch for 10 seconds)
	Repeat 2 to 3 times
Note	— By lifting the head, the abdominal musculature is contracted and the lumbar spine is fixed against the support.

Anterior Hip Muscles

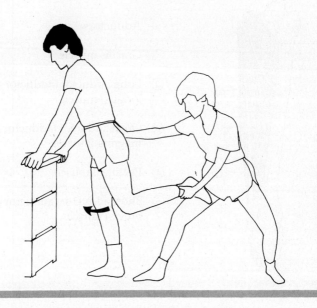

Technique	Dynamic slow strengthening
Execution	← Flex hip
Note	— Your partner provides a stabilizing counterforce against the pelvis.

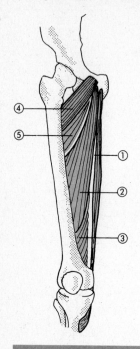

Medial Hip Muscles

Adductors:

① Gracilis muscle

② Long adductor (adductor longus) muscle

③ Great adductor (adductor magnus) muscle

④ Pectineal muscle

⑤ Short adductor (adductor brevis) muscle

Function — Adduction of tigh

Notes — When the hip is flexed more than 30 degrees, the adductors also act as hip flexors. When the hip is extended more than 15 degrees, they support the hip extensors.

— The adductors react tonically and tend to shorten.

— The gracilis muscle is biarticular. Stretching is therefore carried out with the knee extended.

— Problems involving the groin (e. g., among soccer players) are frequently connected with shortening of the adductor musculature.

Medial
Hip Muscles

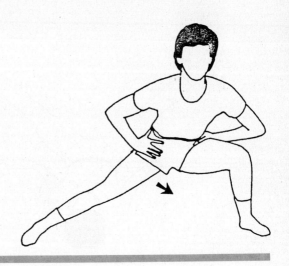

Technique	Passive static stretch
Execution	↘ Push the pelvis obliquely downward
Note	— Easier alternative: the hands are used to support the weight of the trunk on the flexed knee or on the floor.

Medial
Hip Muscles

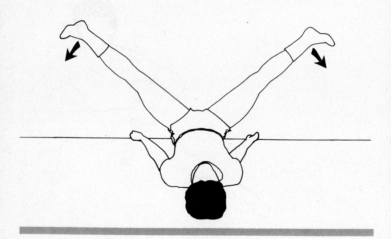

Technique	Passive static stretch
Execution	⚡ Spread the extended legs
Note	— Slide the buttocks as close to the wall as possible.
	— The stretch can be actively increased by pushing with the hands against the inside of the knees.

Medial
Hip Muscles

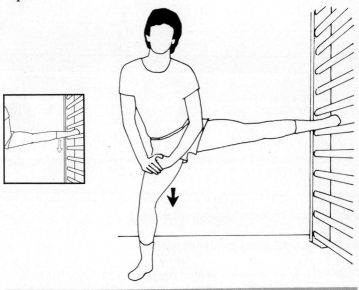

Technique	Contract–relax–stretch
Execution	⇩ Press the leg down onto the rung (3–7 seconds of isometric contraction)
	Relax
	↓ Bend the knee of the upright leg (stretch for 10 seconds)
	Repeat 2 to 3 times
Note	— The stretch is increased if the foot rests on a higher rung.

Medial
Hip Muscles

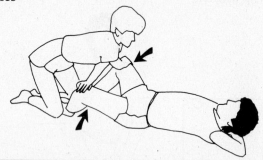

Technique   Dynamic slow strengthening

Execution   ↑↓ Press the thighs together

Note   — To avoid pain in the groin, resistance has to be
          kept within reasonable limits in this exercise.

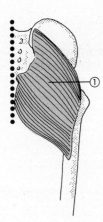

Posterior Hip Muscles

Superficial Layer

① Gluteus maximus muscle

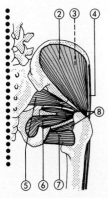

Deep Layer

② Gluteus medius muscle

③ Gluteus minimus muscle (concealed)

④ Tensor fasciae latae muscle

⑤ Piriformis muscle

⑥ External obturator muscle

⑦ Quadratus muscle of the thigh

⑧ Gemellus muscles

Function	— Extension of the hip
①	— External rotation of the thigh
Function	— Abduction of the thigh
② + ③	— Stabilization of the pelvis on the side of the supporting leg against tipping over to the side of the leg being exercised
	— Extension of the hip
	— Internal rotation of the thigh
Function ④	— Abduction of the thigh
Function ⑤ + ⑥ + ⑦ + ⑧	— External rotation of the thigh

Notes
— The gluteus maximus muscle reacts phasically and tends to weaken.
Together with the abdominal musculature and the hamstring (ischiocrural) muscles, it is responsible for the righting of the pelvis. When weakened, the muscle allows the low back to become more arched, which is unfavorable when it is static. This static imbalance is aggravated further when the psoas major, rectus femoris, and erector muscles of the lumbar spine are shortened.

— The gluteus medius and the gluteus minimus muscles also react phasically. Weakening leads to insufficient stabilization of the pelvis.

— The tensor fasciae latae muscle reacts tonically. Its shortening can lead to lateral thigh pain. This occurs particularly if the gluteus medius and minimus muscles are weakened at the same time, for in this situation the tensor fasciae latae muscle is overloaded during stabilization of the pelvis.

— The piriformis muscle is decidedly tonic. Its shortening frequently is responsible for pain deep in the buttocks, which may also radiate toward the posterior aspect of the thigh.

Posterior
Hip Muscles

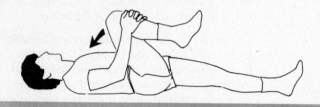

Technique   Passive static stretch

Execution   ✔ Pull knee down

Notes   — The head and the contralateral leg rest on the
                 support.

               — This exercise stretches the hip extensor muscles
                 in particular.

*Posterior
Hip Muscles*

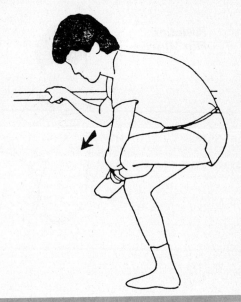

Technique	Passive static stretch
Execution	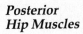 Lean the trunk forward from the waist
Notes	— The stretch is increased by assuming a lower squatting position.
	— Unsteadiness in standing can be avoided by using the other hand for support.

*Posterior
Hip Muscles*

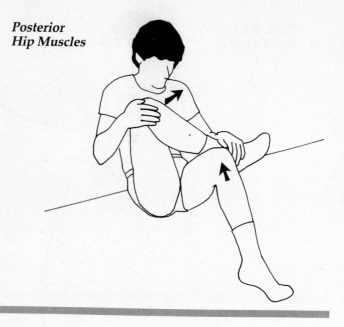

Technique	Passive static stretching
Execution	↑ Press knee against lower leg
	↗ Using your hand, press thigh against the contra-lateral shoulder
Note	— This exercise provides the most intensive stretching of the posterior hip muscles.

Posterior
Hip Muscles

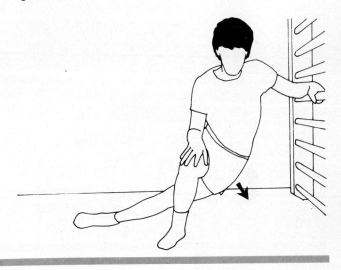

Technique   Passive static stretching

Execution   ↘ Push the pelvis downward

Notes   — Secure stabilization of the trunk is necessary.

            — The principal effect of this stretching exercise is
            exerted on the tensor fasciae latae muscle.

Posterior
Hip Muscles

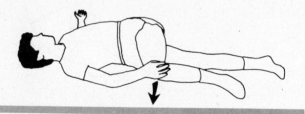

Technique	Passive static stretching
Execution	↓ Pull down the flexed knee with the opposite hand
Notes	— Both shoulders should remain on the floor.
	— This exercise has a mobilizing effect on the lumbar spine and the sacroiliac joints at the same time.

Posterior
Hip Muscles

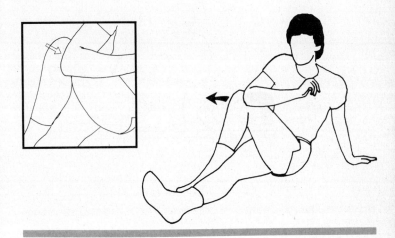

Technique	Contract–relax–stretch
Execution	↘ Press thigh against elbow (isometric contraction for 3–7 seconds)
	Relax
	← Using the elbow, push the thigh to the opposite side (stretch for 10 seconds)
	Repeat 2–3 times
Note	— Depending on the extent of hip flexion, different portions of the posterior hip musculature are stretched.

Posterior Hip Muscles

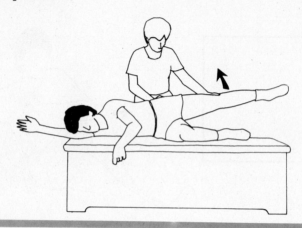

Technique	Dynamic slow strengthening
Execution	↖ Lift the thigh off the table
Notes	— Your partner helps to stabilize the pelvis while you are lying on your side, and checks the plane of motion. Forward or backward movement should be avoided.
	— The chief effect is exerted on the abductors (gluteus medius and minimus and tensor fasciae latae muscles).

Posterior
Hip Muscles

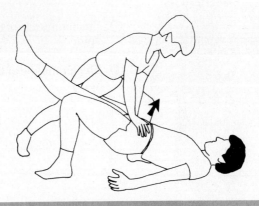

Technique	Dynamic slow strengthening
Execution	↗ Move pelvis upward by extending the hip
Notes	— Below the knee, the supporting leg should be perpendicular to the floor.
	— The back should not be arched.
	— If the gluteal muscles are weak, the exercise may initially be carried out with both legs.
	— This exercise mainly affects the gluteus maximus muscle.

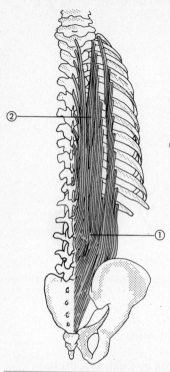

Back Muscles

① Erector muscle of the lumbar spine

② Erector muscle of the thoracic spine

Function

— Extending the vertebral column when the back extensors are contracted bilaterally

— Bending the spine to the side, and rotating it, when the back extensors are contracted unilaterally

— Stabilizing the spine when there is simultaneous contraction of the psoas, major muscle and the abdominal muscles.

Notes
— The back extensors in the lumbar spine react tonically. Shortening leads to increased concavity of the back and is frequently responsible for low back pain.

— The back extensors in the thoracic spine region react phasically and tend to weaken. This is generally associated with increased arching of the back. If the lumbar back extensors shorten at the same time, a lordotic curved back with postural weakness may develop.

— Postural training should include selective strengthening exercises for the erectors of the thoracic spine as well as specific stretching exercises for the lumbar back extensors.

Back Muscles

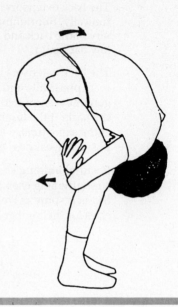

Technique	Passive static stretching
Execution	← Extend the knee
	➤ Increase arching of back
Note	— The exercise is carried out correctly if the stretching is felt primarily in the back muscles, especially in the area of the lumbar spine. It is particularly the lumbar back extensors that need stretching.

Back Muscles

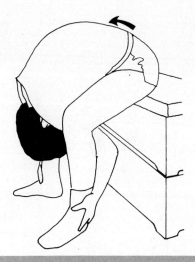

Technique   Passive static stretching

Execution   Increase the rounding of the back by pulling the arms downward.

Note   — If this exercise is carried out correctly, the stretching feeling is experienced in the lumbar spine. The lumbar back extensors should be particularly stretched.

Back Muscles

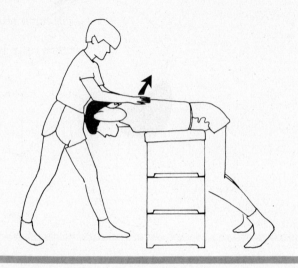

Technique   Dynamic slow strengthening

Execution   ⬈ Extend the back

Notes   — The overall range of motion should remain very
                limited.

              — At the beginning, the weight of the trunk often
                provides enough resistance.

              — Variation: Your partner provides constant resi-
                stance. With the feet raised off the ground, the
                buttocks are slightly raised. Excessive curving
                of the back should be avoided.

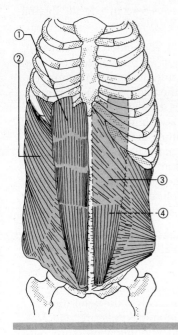

Abdominal Muscles

① Rectus abdominis muscle

② External oblique muscle of the abdomen

③ Internal oblique muscle of the abdomen

④ Transverse muscle of the abdomen (concealed)

Function
— Bending the trunk forward with the pelvis stationary pelvis

— Righting of the pelvis with the chest stationary

— Bending the trunk to the side and rotating it when the abdominal muscles are contracted unilaterally.

— Abdominal pressure

Notes
- The abdominal muscles react in a decidedly phasic manner and tend to weaken.

— A sufficiently strong abdominal musculature, together with the gluteal musculature (see also gluteus maximus) and the hamstring muscles (biceps muscle of the thigh, semimembranous and semitendinous muscles), rights the pelvis. Weakening of the abdominal musculature leads to forward tilting of the pelvis, hence to increased curving of the back. Simultaneous shortening of the lumbar back extensors and the psoas major and rectus femoris muscles increases this lordotic effect, which adversely affects the lumbar spine.

— The abdominal muscles and back muscles function as a dynamic tightening system of the trunk.

— Contraction of the abdominal muscles, the diaphragm, and the muscles of the pelvic floor causes the intra-abdominal pressure to increase. This mechanism (abdominal pressure) permits additional stabilization of the trunk.

— Adequate stabilization of the trunk is of great importance in every sports activity. The strength of the muscles of the arms and legs can only be utilized optimally if the trunk is stable.

Abdominal Muscles

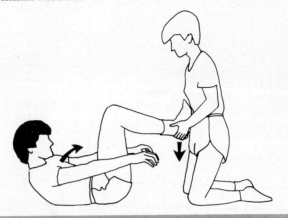

Technique	Dynamic slow strengthening
Execution	↓ Press the heels down
	↗ Raise the upper body, with the lumbar spine resting on the floor
Notes	— This exercise eliminates the action of the hip flexors, thus training the abdominal musculature alone.
	— Care should be taken to maintain regular breathing.

Abdominal Muscles

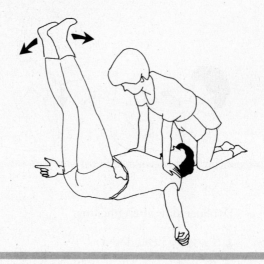

Technique	Dynamic slow strengthening
Execution	Alternately drop and raise legs sideways (windshield wiper motion)
Notes	— The partner provides fixation, particularly on the opposite shoulder.
	— An advanced version of the exercise is carried out with the buttocks off the floor and with an additional load (e. g., medicine ball).

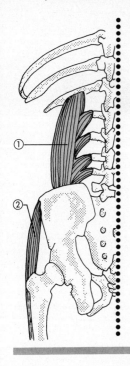

Lateral Trunk Muscles

① Quadratus lumborum muscle

② Tensor fasciae latae muscle

— External oblique muscle of the abdomen

— Internal oblique muscle of the abdomen (see under Abdominal Muscles, p. 77)

Function ①	— Bending the trunk to the side, unilateral contraction
	— Stabilizing the trunk and extending the lumbar spine, with bilateral contraction
Function ②	— Stabilizing the pelvis
	— Abduction of the thigh
Note	— A shortened quadratus lumborum muscle adversely affects the statics of the vertebral column, as it produces increased lordosis. This results in faulty loading of the lumbar spine.

Lateral Trunk Muscles

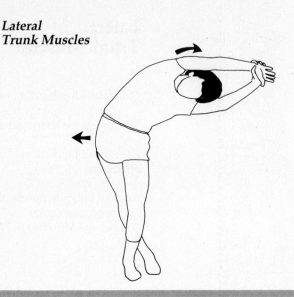

Technique	Passive static stretch
Execution	← Move hip to the side
	➔ Pull trunk to the opposite side
Notes	— Rotation of the upper body (evasive movement) should be avoided
	— When leaning to the left, the left leg should be in front, and vice versa.

Lateral Trunk Muscles

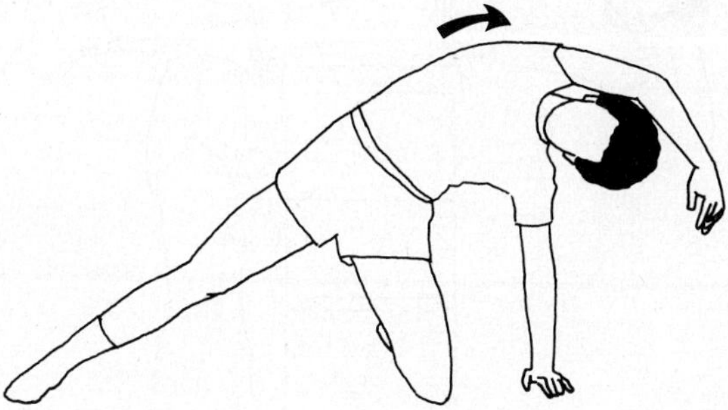

Technique Passive static stretch

Execution ➔ Bend the trunk to one side at the waist

Note — The trunk should make a purely lateral movement, without any deviation forward or backward.

Lateral
Trunk Muscles

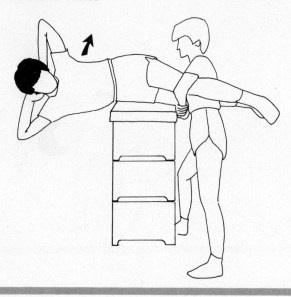

Technique	Dynamic slow strengthening
Execution	↑ Raise the trunk sideways
Notes	— Your partner holds you in place at the thighs.
	— The partner monitors the movement. To strengthen the lateral trunk musculature only, the trunk should not rotate.
	— If the exercise is carried out with rotation of the trunk, the oblique abdominal muscles are strengthened as well.

Chest Muscles

① Pectoralis major muscle

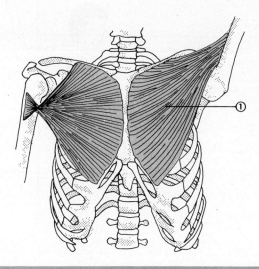

Function
— Forward flexion of the arm

— Adduction of the laterally raised arm

— Internal rotation of the upper arm

— Stabilization of the shoulder joint in conjunction with the other shoulder muscles

— Support of inspiration when the arms are resting on the elbows

Note
— A bilaterally shortened chest musculature produces a forward-leaning posture by pulling the shoulders forward. The fixator muscles of the shoulder-blades (rhomboid muscles) and the back extensor muscles in the thoracic spine are often weakened at the same time ("postural weakness").

Chest Muscles

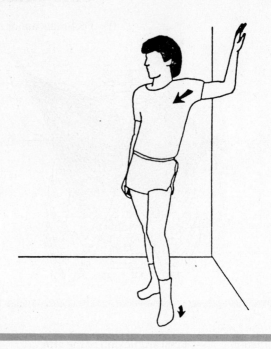

Technique	Passive static stretch
Execution	↓ Take a step forward with the leg on the same side
	↙ Move your shoulder forward
Note	— Holding the arm higher and lower allows the different portions of the pectoralis major muscle to be stretched.

Chest Muscles

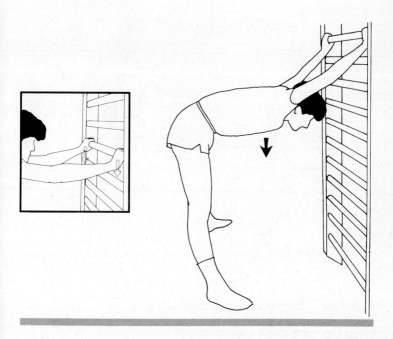

Technique	Contract–relax–stretch
Execution	⇓⇓ Press your arms downward (3–7 seconds of isometric contraction)
	Relax
	↓ Press the upper body downward and exhale (10-second stretch)
	Repeat 2–3 times
Note	— By varying the distance between the hands, different parts of the chest musculature are stretched.

Chest Muscles

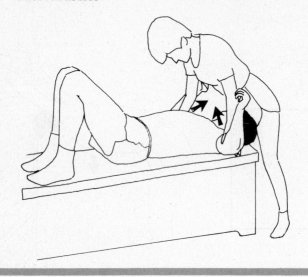

Technique   Dynamic slow strengthening

Execution   ↗↖ Press arms forward

Notes   — Your partner creates resistance at a point just
             above the elbow joints.

          — The entire range of motion should be utilized.

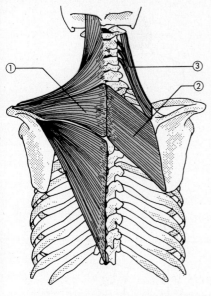

Shoulder Girdle Muscles

① Trapezius muscle

② Rhomboid major and minor muscles

③ Levator scapulae muscle

Function
— Raising the shoulder girdle

— Pulling the shoulder blades toward the spine (shoulder blade fixation)

— Stabilizing the cervical spine

— Support for inspiration

Notes
— Weak rhomboid muscles fix the shoulder blades inadequately. The shoulders are consequently pulled forward by the chest muscles. A bent-over posture in the upper body (hunchback) usually results.

— Pain in the back of the neck is often associated with simultaneous weakening of the shoulder blade fixators and shortening of the levator scapulae muscle as well as the descending portion of the trapezius muscle.

Shoulder Girdle Muscles

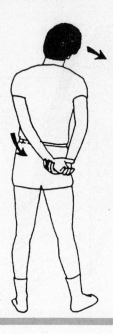

Technique	Passive static stretching
Execution	↘ Lean your head toward the opposite side
	↘ Pull your arm downward and exhale
Note	— The upper body should be straight. Avoid turning the head.

Shoulder Girdle Muscles

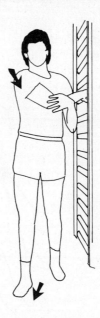

Technique	Passive static stretching
Executing	↓ Take a step forward with the leg on the same side
	↘ Press the upper body forward
Note	— The upper body should continue to lean forward and an evasive shift into a hollow-back position should be avoided.

Shoulder Girdle Muscles

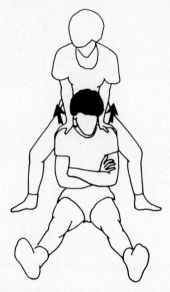

Technique   Dynamic slow strengthening

Execution   ↑↑ Raise both shoulders

Note   — An upright seated position should be maintained.

Shoulder Girdle Muscles

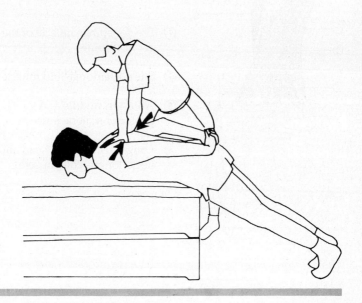

Technique	Dynamic slow strengthening
Execution	Draw shoulder blades toward one another
Note	— With arms crossed your partner provides resistance against both shoulder-blades.

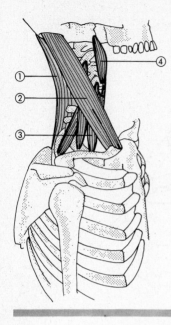

Neck Muscles

① Erector spinae muscle of the cervical spine

② Sternocleidomastoid muscle

③ Anterior, middle and posterior scalene muscles

④ Long muscle of the head and neck (longus colli muscle)

Function
①

— Extension (bending the head backward), with bilateral contraction

— Turning the head toward the contracting side, with unilateral contraction

Function
②③④

Flexion (bending the head forward), with bilateral contraction

– Bending the head to the side, with unilateral contraction

— Turning the head to the opposite side, with unilateral contraction

— Supporting inspiration (scalene muscles, sternocleidomastoid muscle)

Notes

— The erector spinae muscle of the cervical spine consists of a large number of small muscles.

— In sport activities (e. g., when wearing a helmet, football), good stabilization of the cervical spine is essential. Weakened muscles may cause strain symptoms.

— Shortened neck muscles produce malpositioning of the cervical spine and consequently cause reduced exercise tolerance and increased susceptibility to injury.

Neck Muscles

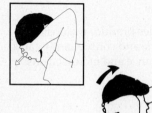

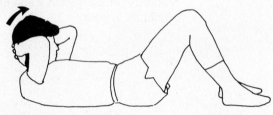

Technique	Contract–relax–stretch
Execution	Press your head backward and inhale (3–7 seconds of isometric contraction)
	Relax
	Pull your head forward with both hands and exhale (stretch for 10 seconds) Repeat 2–3 times
Notes	— Pulling the head forward should be combined with longitudinal traction ("pulling the head out of the neck").
	— This exercise often proves beneficial when there is pain in the back of the neck and headache.
	— If dizziness occurs, the exercise should be terminated immediately.
	— In view of the appreciable load on the intervertebral disks and ligaments, this exercise should not be done in the first few weeks after a sprain of the cervical spine.

Neck Muscles

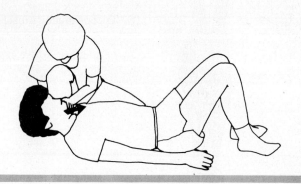

Technique	Dynamic slow strengthening
Execution	↗ Nodding movement of the head
Notes	— Your partner provides resistance at the chin.
	— The nodding movement is performed only in the upper cervical spine. The lower cervical spine should not be flexed.

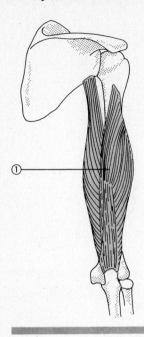

Posterior Arm Muscles

① Triceps brachii muscle

Function	— Stretching of the elbow joint
Note	— The long head of the triceps brachii muscle is biarticular. Acting on the shoulder joint, it causes the raised arm to be drawn downward and backward (used in throwing and in cross-country skiing).

Posterior
Arm Muscles

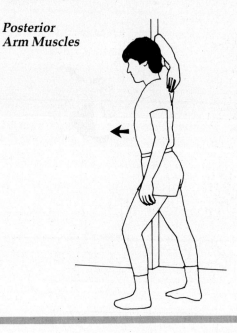

Technique	Passive static stretch
Execution	← With the arm secured in a raised position with the elbow flexed, move the trunk forward
Note	— This is an important stretching exercise for sports activities involving frequent overhead movements (tennis, volleyball, throwing contests).

*Posterior
Arm Muscles*

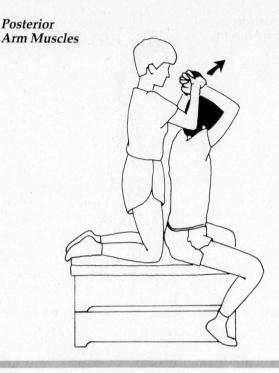

Technique	Dynamic slow strengthening
Execution	➚ Extend both elbows
Notes	— Keep your back as straight as possible.
	— As always, the full range of motion should be utilized.

Anterior Arm Muscles

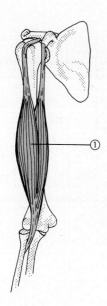

① Biceps brachii muscle

Function	— Flexion of the elbow joint
	— Supination of the forearm (upward rotation of palm)
Notes	— The biceps muscle is a biarticular muscle. The long head supports abduction and internal rotation in the shoulder joint, while the short head supports adduction. In conjunction with the other shoulder muscles, the biceps muscle stabilizes the shoulder joint.
	— Two other muscles act as flexors in the elbow joint: the brachial muscle and the brachioradialis muscle.

Anterior Arm Muscles

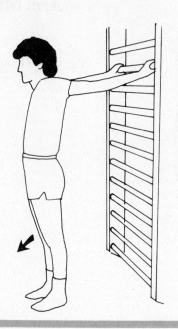

Technique	Passive static stretch
Execution	✔ Move your trunk downward and forward by bending the knees
Notes	— The stretch has to be kept within limits to avoid undue tension on the joint capsules and ligaments associated with the shoulder joint.

Anterior Arm Muscles

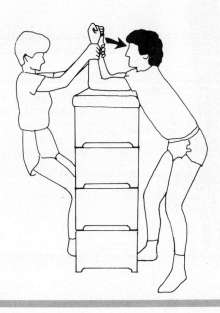

Technique	Dynamic slow strengthening
Execution	➤ Bend your elbows
Notes	— The arms must not be lifted off their support.
	— The full range of motion should be utilized, if possible.

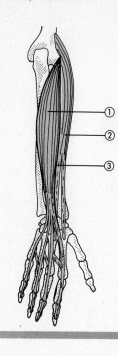

Lateral Forearm Muscles

① Extensor digitorum muscle (extensor muscle of fingers)

② Extensor carpi radialis longus muscle (long radial extensor muscle of the wrist)

① Extensor carpi radialis brevis muscle (short radial extensor muscle of the wrist)

Function — Extension of the fingers

— Dorsal extension of the wrist ("cocking up" of wrist).

— Stabilization of the wrist, together with the flexor muscles

Note — The extensor musculature originates at the lateral epicondyle of the humerus. Tendon insertion disorders (e. g., "tennis elbow") at this site can often be alleviated or even avoided by selective stretching of these muscles.

Lateral Forearm Muscles

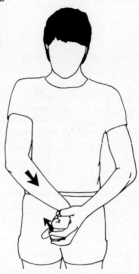

Technique	Passive static stretch
Execution	↖ Hold your hand with the wrist and finger joints bent
	↘ Extend the elbow
Note	— The muscle stretching is more effective when the wrist and finger joints are kept bent as much as possible.

Lateral Forearm Muscles

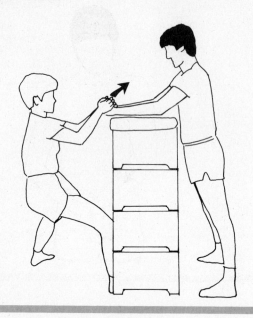

Technique	Dynamic slow strengthening
Execution	↗ Extend wrists
Notes	— Your partner provides resistance at the back of the hand.
	— The forearms rest on the support.
	— The movement should range from full flexion of the wrist to full extension.

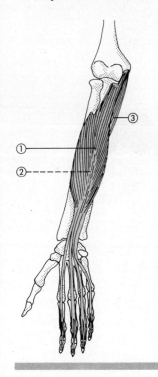

Medial Forearm Muscles

① Flexor digitorum superficialis muscle (superficial flexor muscle of the fingers)

② Flexor digitorum profundus muscle (deep flexor muscle of the fingers, concealed)

③ Flexor carpi radialis muscle (radial flexor muscle of the wrist)

Function
— Flexion of the fingers

— Flexion at the wrist (bending the wrist)

— Stabilization of the wrist, together with the extensor muscles

Note
— The flexor musculature originates at the medial epicondyle of the humerus. Tendon insertion disorders ("pitchers' elbow," "golfers' elbow") may be alleviated by stretching the flexor muscles. Great value is attached to prophylactic stretching.

Medial Forearm Muscles

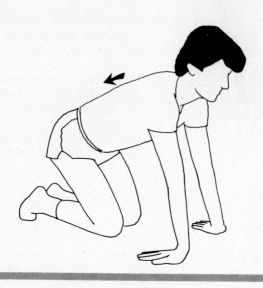

Technique	Passive static stretch
Execution	✔ Move the trunk backward
Note	— The more the hands are turned backward, the better the stretch.

Medial
Forearm Muscles

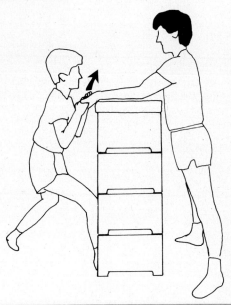

Technique	Dynamic slow strengthening
Execution	↗ Bend your wrists
Notes	— Your partner provides resistance at the palms.
	— Your forearms rest on the support.
	— The full range of motion should be utilized, if possible.

Theoretical Principles

Muscular Imbalance

On the basis of their developmental history, the different muscles can be divided into three groups according to function:

— Tonic musculature
— Mixed musculature
— Phasic musculature

The tonic musculature originally had a purely postural function, while movement was the main function of the phasic musculature. Muscle groups that have both functions are described as mixed musculature.

In man, tonic and phasic muscles are no longer found in their pure form. Nonetheless, certain muscles can be assigned to one or the other muscle group according to their response to faulty loading or overloading. The predominantly tonic muscles react by *shortening,* and the predominantly phasic muscles by *weakening* (Table 1).

There is, however, a direct relationship between these two muscle groups in that a shortened tonic muscle can inhibit its phasic antagonists and synergists, thus preventing their maximal activation and optimal trainability.

Most muscles are neutral with regard to shortening and weakening (mixed musculature). Table 2 lists those muscles which have a *predominantly* tonic or phasic reaction.

Table 1   Properties of tonic and phasic musculature

	Tonic	Phasic
Function	Posture	Movement
Innervation	α-2-motoneuron	α-1-motoneuron
Susceptibility to fatigue	Late	Early
Reaction to faulty loading	Shortening	Weakening

Table **2** Classification of muscles

Predominantly tonic muscles	Predominantly phasic muscles
Shoulder girdle–Arm	
Pectoralis major muscle	Rhomboid muscles
Levator scapulae muscle	Trapezius muscle (ascending part)
Trapezius muscle (descending part)	Trapezius muscle (horizontal part)
Biceps brachii muscle	
Scalene muscles	Triceps brachii muscle
Trunk	
Erector muscles of the lumbar and cervical spine	Erector muscle of the middle thoracic spine
Quadratus lumborum muscle	Abdominal muscles
Pelvis–Thigh	
Biceps muscle of the thigh	Vastus medialis muscle
Semitendinous muscle	Vastus lateralis muscle
Semimembranous muscle	
Iliopsoas muscle	Gluteus medius muscle
Rectus femoris muscle	Gluteus maximus muscle
	Gluteus minimus muscle
Long adductor muscle	
Short adductor muscle	
Great adductor muscle	
Gracilis muscle	
Piriformis muscle	
Tensor fasciae latae muscle	
Lower Leg–Foot	
Gastrocnemius muscle	Anterior tibialis muscle
Soleus muscle	Peroneal muscle

Muscular imbalance is a condition in which there is a lack of balance between the tonic and the phasic musculature. While strength is retained, the tonic muscles are *shortened;* the phasic antagonists and synergists show a *weakening* at normal length.

This *shortening* and *weakening* can easily be clinically assessed by specific length and strength testing.

In sports activities, the most common cause of muscular imbalance is faulty loading or overloading of the locomotor system. Frequently, injuries or other pathologic processes involving the locomotor system (wear and tear, inflammation, etc.) may be the precipitating factors. Whithout appropriate stretching and strengthening exercises, unfavorable conditions can persist for a long time (Fig. 5).

Several studies have shown that these episodes of muscular imbalance are common among athletes. Many of the athletes studied were found to have more or less pronounced muscle shortening and muscle weakening. The prime reasons were unilateral, faulty, and excessive exercise.

Muscular imbalance reduces the exercise tolerance of the locomotor apparatus. Shortened tonic muscles go into action more rapidly to produce defensive and protective movements than do phasic muscles. This can lead to short-term mechanical overloading and the risk of muscle strains or even tears in the shortened tonic musculature. Shortened muscles are less supple and less elastic in the relaxation phase. This increased internal resistance often causes a painful overloading of the affected muscles and tendons. Regional muscular imbalance puts increased stress on joints and spinal segments, causing states of irritation.

The goal in the treatment of muscular imbalance is the abolition of shortening and weakening (see Fig. **4,** p. 5).

Selective exercises should therefore stretch certain muscles, on the one hand, while strengthening others: *stretching and strengthening exercises.* Stretching, taken in the narrow sense, lacks the element of selective strengthening. Both factors are necessary, however, to relieve muscular imbalance.

It should be borne in mind that optimal strengthening of shortened muscle groups is possible only if the shortened muscles have been stretched to their normal length first: *stretching comes before strengthening.*

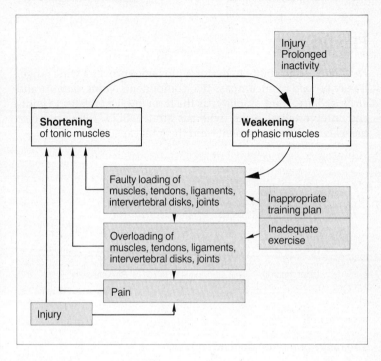

Fig. **5**   Muscular imbalance

Flexibility

Flexibility is the ability to perform movements over a wide range.
It may be said to encompass two components, *joint mobility* and
stretchability. Joint mobility, as the term implies, relates to joints
and intervertebral disks, whereas stretchability refers more to
muscles, tendons, ligaments and the joint capsules.

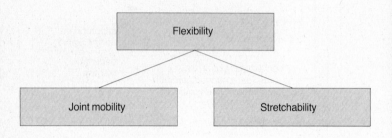

The range of motion depends on:

— the shape of the joint surfaces involved and the degree of
  freedom of the individual joint:
— the stretchability of the muscles, tendons, ligaments and
  joint capsules;
— the strength of the musculature.

Active motion refers to the range of motion in a joint attainable
by the intrinsic muscular force (physiologic range of motion).
When the maximal range of motion, up to the limit of anatomical
mobility, is produced by external forces (examiner, partner,
gravity, equipment), we refer to *passive motion.* The passive
range of motion is always greater than the active one (Fig. **6**).

  Active and passive motion may be increased beyond the
normal range, leading to reduced stability of the vertebral
column and joints. This in turn poses a serious risk of injury.

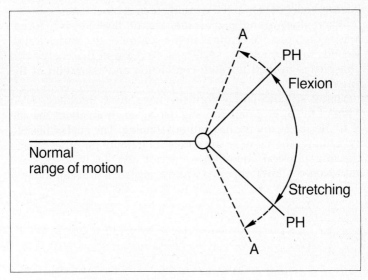

Fig. 6 Normal flexibility of joints

PH physiologic limit of mobility
A   anatomical limit of mobility

The range of motion (flexibility) is directly influenced by a whole series of external factors:

With *increasing age,* stretchability, and thus flexibility, diminishes owing to chemical and structural changes in the muscles and tendons. These aging processes lead to a decrease of elastic fibers, loss of water, and a reduction in the number and activity of cells. When degenerative changes occur in a joint (osteoarthritis), the range of motion is reduced by changes in the articular architecture.

Hormonal differences account for the fact that women's muscles, tendons and ligaments are more stretchable.

The *temperature* of the active locomotor system directly affects flexibility. A rise in temperature due to active warming (warm-up) or passive warming (increased ambient temperature, hot bath, etc.) improves stretchability. Active warming is preferable to passive warming. Thus, an adequate warm-up should be part of any flexibility training.

Flexibility is subject to *variation* during the course of the day. It is markedly poorer in the morning than at other times.

When *physical* and *mental fatigue* occur, flexibility is reduced. This is due, first, to changes in the control of the muscles and, second, to local factors, such as a decrease in the energy-rich phosphates needed for both contraction and relaxation of the muscles.

Young schoolchildren normally have good flexibility, even without the appropriate training. However, from about the age of 10, flexibility diminishes without training. The goal of flexibility training, therefore — in contrast to training for other factors affecting physical condition — is not necessarily to produce improvement, but rather to prevent a "negative" development.

The Muscle — Structure and Properties

Skeletal musculature accounts for 40–50% of total body weight. The musculature is thus by far the largest organ in man. Its main function is to generate force. The contraction this requires is made possible by the specific *microstructure of the muscle* (Fig. 7).

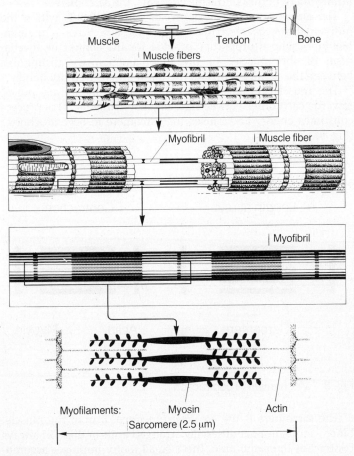

Fig. 7   Structure of muscle

Normal skeletal muscle consists of a muscle belly and the tendons adjoining it at each end, which are anchored in the bone. The basic unit of the muscle is the muscle fiber. This may range from a few to several centimeters in length, depending on the particular muscle. The individual muscle fibers are joined to muscle bundles by elastic and nonelastic connective-tissue fibers. The muscle fibers are composed of a large number of myofibrils, which have a striated pattern when seen under the light microscope. This cross-striation is produced by the regular arrangement of the contractile elements, the *sarcomeres.*

The electron microscope preveals further details within the individual sarcomeres. These are protein structures — myofilaments — whose properties provide for the contractile mechanism of the muscle. In the myofilaments, we distinguish between the slender *actin* and the thicker *myosin* components.

The muscle contracts when the actin filaments are pulled towards each other between the myosin filaments. This process consumes energy and causes the sarcomere to become shorter (Fig. 8).

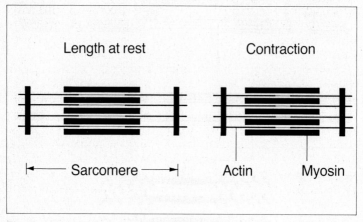

Fig. 8   Mechanism of contraction

The sarcomere is the *smallest functional unit* of the muscle. Since a large number of serially arranged units of this sort always contract at the same time, these small motor impulses accumulate into a larger movement.

Two different *types of muscle fibers* can be distinguished on the basis of the differing contents of enzymes for energy supply (e. g., myosin ATPase), the structure of the myosin filaments, and the type of innervation (impulse pattern of motoneurons):

Fiber Type I ("slow twitch", ST or red fibers):

These fibers are characterized by their slower rate of contraction, by their aerobic metabolism with the relevant enzymes, and high resistance to fatigue. Tonic muscles normally contain a higher percentage of this type of fiber. As a rule, highly trained endurance athletes, such as cyclists, long-distance runners, and cross-country skiers, have a larger proportion of Type I fibers.

Fiber Type II ("fast twitch", FT or white fibers)

These fibers are distinguished by their higher rate of contraction, their anaerobic metabolism, and low resistance to fatigue. Phasic muscles contain a higher percentage of Type II fibers. Both maximal strength and rapid strength development are directly related to the percentage of this fiber type present in muscle. Sprinters, weight-lifters, and long jumpers and high jumpers, for example, have a large proportion of Type II fibers.

The individual distribution of these two fiber types is partly inborn, and partly dependent on the type of stress to which the musculature is subjected. Transformation of Type II fibers into Type I fibers can be accomplished far more readily through endurance training than, conversely, the transformation of Type I fibers into Type II fibers can through strength or interval training. This is why a good long-distance runner can hardly ever become a good sprinter. By contrast, a sprinter can significantly improve his long-distance performance at the expense of his speed.

Owing to their special composition, with contractile elements (sarcomeres) and connective tissue components, muscles have *contractile* as well as *elastic* properties. The tendons, consisting of taut connective tissue, have only a low degree of elasticity. It is a common characteristic of both structures that they can be deformed to a certain extent, thus exhibiting *plastic* behavior:

when a muscle or a tendon is relaxed after a period of stretching, an increase in length — "residual stretch" — persists for some time.

When a muscle, tendon, or ligament is stretched beyond its physiologic limits, the structure is injured. These physiologic limits should be borne in mind during flexibility training.

The Muscle and Muscle Control

The musculature has two functions:

1. Maintaining posture
2. Executing movement

A sophisticated system of control and regulation is needed to allow the muscles to meet these two different requirements. These control processes may by represented as a control circuit (Fig. 9).

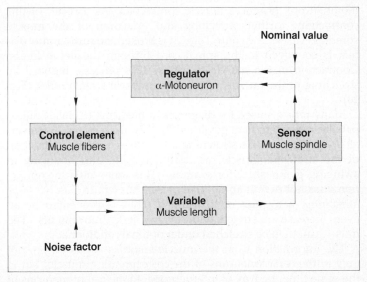

Fig. 9   Muscle control system

The *posture function* requires that the muscle be able to keep its length constant despite the impingement of external forces. The muscle length is measured by a sensor *(muscle spindle)* and the information obtained in this way is relayed to a regulator *(motoneuron* in the spinal cord). This regulator performs the necessary correction of the length via the muscle fibers.

A similar system is required to control the *movement function* of the musculature. This system must be able to adapt to varying muscle length and muscle tension, and this adaptability is accomplished through continuous adjustment of the nominal value.

To measure muscle length and tension, both the muscles and the corresponding tendons have special sensors (receptors). In the muscles, these are the *muscle spindles;* in the tendons, they are the *Golgi tendon organs.*

The *muscle spindles,* arranged in parallel to the muscle fibers, record changes in muscle length. This information is passed on to the corresponding α-motoneurons in the anterior horn of the spinal cord via fast-conducting nerve fibers. Stimulation of these motoneurons produces muscle contraction. As a result of this contraction, further stretching and excitation of the muscle spindles ceases. The control circuit is broken; no further information is conveyed to the spinal cord through the nerve fibers. Contraction of the muscle subsides. This process, induced by stretching of the muscle, is called the muscle *stretch reflex* (Fig. 10).

Many reflexes used for diagnosis in medicine (Achilles reflex, patellar reflex, etc.) are governed by this mechanism. However, all short-term muscle stretching also causes a reflex contraction of the stretched muscle, as during rocking and bouncing in swinging gymnastics, for example. This reflex muscle contraction does not permit an optimal muscle stretch. In *passive static stretching,* activation of the stretch reflex is prevented by an even increase of stretch without any jerky movements. The muscle can then be stretched under optimal conditions.

The information from the muscle spindles is passed on, not only to the α-motoneurons of the corresponding muscle, but at the same time, by way of interneurons, to the α-motoneurons of its antagonists. These motoneurons, and consequently their antagonists as well, are inhibited: *reciprocal inhibition of the antagonists* occurs.

Thus, when a flexor muscle is contracted, the corresponding extensor muscle is relaxed, and upon activation of the extensor, the corresponding flexors are relaxed. This mechanism for muscle relaxation is used in *active static stretching.*

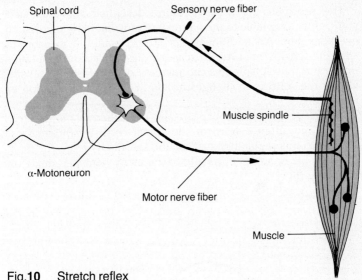

Fig.10 Stretch reflex

The *Golgi tendon organs* are located at the junction between muscle and tendon. They are stimulated when the tension rises sharply in the muscle, the tendon. This information, too, is transmitted via nerve fibers and interneurons to the α-motoneurons in the spinal cord. These motoneurons are *inhibited,* and the muscle contraction is diminished. Relaxation of the muscle and the tendon results. This process is called *self-inhibition.*

Self-inhibition, together with other neurophysiologic processes at the level of the spinal cord, accounts for the phenomenon of *postisometric inhibition.* This involves a short-lived muscle relaxation following isometric contraction of the muscle. This relaxation phase may be utilized for optimal stretching of this muscle — *contract–relax–stretch.*

The processes for muscle control described above are not sufficiently adaptable to the patterns of movement demanded by everyday life. An additional mechanism makes it possible to alter the sensitivity of the muscle spindles. Special muscle fibers *inside* the muscle spindles can increase or decrease the sensitivity of the sensors to changes in length through contraction or relaxation.

These special muscle fibers are also controlled by motor nerve cells in the anterior horn of the spinal cord: γ-motoneurons. Thanks to this regulatory system, the so-called γ-loop, the muscles are able to adjust optimally to the many demands made on them (Fig. 11).

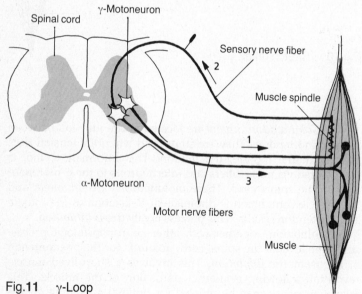

Fig.11   γ-Loop

1 Activation of muscle fibers within the muscle spindle by the γ-moto-neuron.
2 Feedback of changes in the length of the muscle spindle to the α-motoneuron via the sensory nerve fiber. The α-motoneuron is stimulated.
3 The impulse is transmitted to the muscle via the motor nerve fiber. As a result, a muscle contraction is induced.

Muscle control, of course, does not take place exclusively at the level of the spinal cord and muscle. Presumably, only the reflex processes used in the various stretching techniques occur at this level, which is subordinate to various brain centers that exert activating or inhibiting effects.

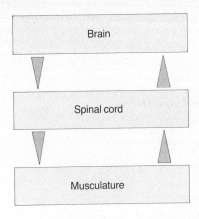

The motor cortex of the brain is responsible chiefly for voluntary movements, while the brain stem is responsible for involuntary movements. These centers in turn are linked to other brain structures, so that — and this is very important in this context — an individual's current state of mind, for example, also affects the state of tension in the musculature. This point should certainly be taken into consideration in stretching exercises.

How to Stretch

We can distinguish basically between two methods of stretching exercises. One consists of bounce-stretching exercises — *dynamic stretching* — and the other is slow stretching — *static stretching*. In the static method, we distinguish between passive static stretching exercises and neuromuscular stretching exercises.

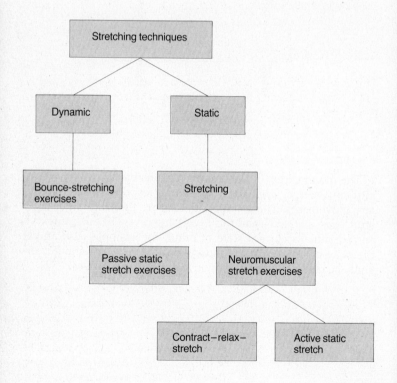

Dynamic Stretching Technique

Dynamic stretching is the type that is still practiced most frequently in current gymnastics activities. An attempt is made to stretch the muscles as much as possible and to extend the range of joint motion by bouncing, rocking, and swinging. The jerky, short-lived muscle stretch leads to the stretch reflex being induced. This reflex causes an immediate muscle contraction which counteracts the attempt to stretch. This neurophysiologic mechanism thus prevents optimal stretching of the musculature. This method of traditional sports exercise is therefore not included in the practical examples of exercises given here.

Static Stretching Techniques

This type of stretching can either be carried out entirely passively or by using neuromuscular processes to achieve complete relaxation of the muscle that is to be stretched.

Passive Static Stretching Exercises

In purely passive static stretching — the best-known form of stretching — the stretch position is assumed, and the muscle is then stretched further by a small change from this position. This change of position can be effected by gravity, one's own muscular force, a partner, or an appliance. If the antagonist alone is used with one's own muscular force, it is equivalent to the active static stretching described below.

A change in the stretch position brings about a gradual increase in resistance. The position at which the feeling of stretch is still tolerable is maintained. A slight pulling in the muscle is permitted, but there should be no pain. Pain would mean that the stretching was unduly intense and harmful. The appropriate feeling of tension can only be judged when some experience has been gained. Stretching therefore has to be learnt. Its intensity needs to be chosen individually. Stretching is *not* a competitive activity.

The goal of slow stretching is to avoid activating the stretch reflex, whenever possible. In this way, the stretch can be applied to a relaxed muscle, without being disturbed by reflex muscle contractions.

Recommendations about the duration of the stretch phase vary between seconds and minutes. A duration of 15–30 seconds is sufficient for effective stretching.

The normal respiratory rate should be retained during the stretch phase. The musculature can be optimally stretched only if adequate attention is also paid to general relaxation.

Neuromuscular Stretching Exercises

In this method of stretching, deliberate use is made of the neurophysiologic processes to achieve muscle relaxation. The stretching can thus be done under the best possible conditions. Both *postisometric inhibition,* on the one hand, and *reciprocal inhibition of the antagonists,* on the other, are utilized. These neurophysiologic mechanisms are described in greater detail on pages 124 and 125.

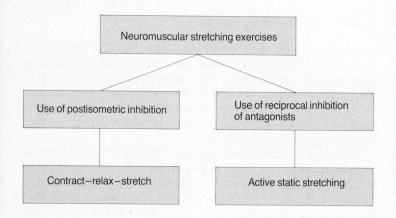

Contract–Relax–Stretch

Starting from the stretched position, the muscle is isometrically contracted for 3–7 seconds. During the muscle relaxation phase following this contraction *(postisometric inhibition),* the stretch position — just as in passive static stretching — is increased and maintained for 10 seconds. Starting from this new stretch position, the whole sequence is repeated: isometric contraction, followed by relaxation, and finally stretching.

This form of stretching is used in therapy when a shortened muscle is to be stretched to its normal length. For a healthy athlete's daily exercise, passive static stretching is sufficient to maintain normal muscle length.

Active Static Stretching

The muscle to be stretched is *actively* brought into a stretched position by contracting its antagonists. This results in reflex inhibition *(reciprocal inhibition)* of the muscle concerned. Because of the muscular relaxation this produces, an optimal stretch can be carried out. The stretch phase lasts 10–20 seconds.

When to Stretch

Generally speaking, stretching exercises should be involved in preparation for any sports activity; they are also an important regenerative measure to be included in the final down-training program, and they undoubtedly belong in any flexibility training. In addition, daily exercises — in the morning after getting up, at the workplace, or at various other times during the day — will consist for the most part of stretching exercises.

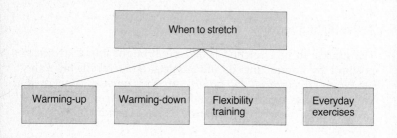

The *intensity* of the stretching depends on the particular situation. It will be greater with warmed-up muscles than with cold or fatigued ones.

Before starting a stretching exercise routine or a flexibility training program, the muscles and tendons should be warmed up actively by running, hopping, cycling, or similar exercises.

Careful, proportionate stretching exercises are among the most important *regenerative (relaxation) measures* to be carried out at the conclusion of physical exertion.The purpose of this is to return the fatigued musculature to its normal length, not to obtain any additional improvement in flexibility. Increased flexibility can be accomplished by those stretching exercises that form part of a general flexibility training program, not when the muscles are fatigued. After intense physical exercise, muscle stretching should be done only with great care, even on the days following the intense activity.

The importance of stretching after strength training has been clearly shown in a Swedish study: in strength training of the legs without subsequent stretching exercises, the range of motion of the major joints of the lower extremities remained restricted for 2–3 days. However, if the muscles in question were stretched immediately after the strength training, the range of motion remained normal (Möller 1981).

Stretching exercises lasting 15 minutes, 2–3 times a week, should be included in the training program. For more intensive training, frequency and duration are increased accordingly. Only *regular* stretching will yield the desired results.

Stretching is less suitable as a direct preparation for competition. In order to maintain the proper basal tone of the musculature and to ensure the range of motion needed in competitive sports, the musculature needs to be stretched dynamically as well (goal-directed exercises).

Recently injured muscles must *not* be stretched so long as there is a danger that the effects of the injury will be exacerbated.

The time to resume an adjusted and carefully proportioned stretching exercise program has to be decided by the physician or therapist. In case of ligament injuries, great care has to be taken to choose stretch exercises that do not stress the injured structure.

Injury to the locomotor apparatus, however, should *never* cause exercises to be discontinued entirely. Only the injured parts of the body must be excluded from stretching exercises. The other parts function normally and should continue to be normally exercised through *compensatory training* so that the level of performance previously reached may be maintained, if at all possible. Early and safe resumption of sports activity is only possible in this way.

How to Strengthen

Basics

Every muscle contraction produces strength. This strength can be used to overcome or counteract resistance. Depending on the force and duration of the strength developed, three types may be distinguished:

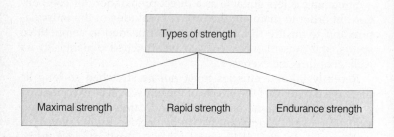

Maximal strength represents the greatest possible force that can be voluntarily opposed to a resistance. It depends on the muscle cross-section and on intramuscular coordination. The *muscle cross-section* is determined by the number and thickness of the muscle fibers. *Intramuscular coordination* relates to nervous control of the musculature. A maximal development of strength is achieved if the individual muscle fibers within a muscle contract simultaneously.

Rapid strength refers to the ability to develop strength almost instantaneously and to maintain it throughout the range of motion. One's own body, limbs, or equipment, are thus moved at a high rate of speed. Rapid strength is chiefly dependent on intramuscular coordination.

Endurance strength denotes the fatigue resistance to long-lasting or repetitive applications of strength. It is determined by maximal strength and anaerobic endurance.

Muscular work can be overriding *(concentric),* or elastic *(eccentric),* or persistent, or it may include a combination of these characteristics.

Depending on the conditions under which the muscle contracts, we speak of *isometric, isotonic* or *auxotonic* forms of contraction. These terms are derived from the type of change in muscle length and muscle tension that is taking place in each case.

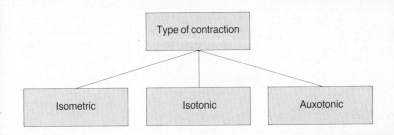

In *isometric* muscle contraction, the muscle length remains constant but muscle tension changes. A muscle contraction is *isotonic* if the muscular tension remains the same throughout the range of motion and only muscle length changes. In *auxotonic* muscle contraction, both muscle tone and muscle length change.

Strength Training

Methods of strength training can be subdivided into dynamic and static types. *Dynamic strength training* means that the training involves movement. In *static strength training,* work at rest or against resistance is carried out without movement.

The following are the most common methods of strength training:

Dynamic rapid strength training: Individual repetition of the exercises is performed with high to maximal use of strength. This method of dynamic rapid strength training can improve all types of strength. The number of repetitions and the loading should vary according to the desired training effect (Table **3**).

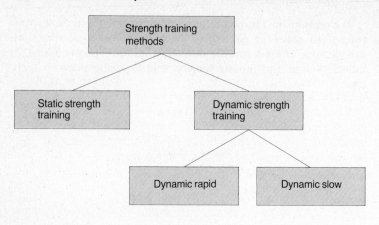

Table 3   Strength training methods, areas of application, number of repetitions, and load

Strength training method	Area of application	Repe- titions	Load %
Dynamic rapid	Maximal strength		
	– intramuscular coordination	1– 5	85–100
	– muscle cross-section	6– 12	70– 85
	Rapid strength	10– 15	30– 60
	Endurance strength	20– 60	30– 50
Dynamic slow (isokinetic)	Maximal strength		
	– muscle cross-section	8– 12	50– 70
	Endurance strength	10– 20	30– 50
Static (isometric)	Maximal strength		
	– intramuscular coordination	3– 5 s	90–100
	– muscle cross-section	6– 10 s	70– 90
	Endurance strength	30–120 s	30– 50

s: seconds

Dynamic slow strength training: Movements are slow and even (proportionate use, of strength). This training method is also called isokinetic strength training. Dynamic slow strength training is suitable for increasing muscle cross-section and endurance (Table 3). It is not suited for improving rapid strength.

Static strength training: Maximal static or isometric development of strength against fixed resistance improves static maximal strength. To improve static endurance, use is made of a submaximal muscle contraction for prolonged duration (Table 3). Static strength training is of secondary importance in most types of sports because it does not involve movement and does not promote coordination. It is most likely to be beneficial in training the trunk musculature because of the trunk muscles' combination of postural and motor functions.

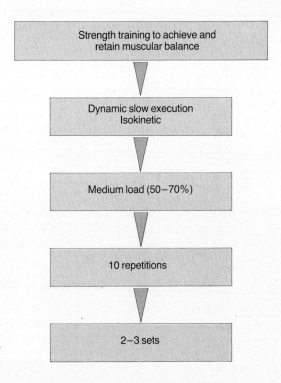

Strength training to achieve and retain muscular balance

Dynamic slow execution Isokinetic

Medium load (50–70%)

10 repetitions

2–3 sets

Dynamic slow (isokinetic) strength training is best suited for the attainment and maintenance of muscular balance. Each training unit encompasses 2–3 series of 10 repetitions with an average load of 50–70%. This produces an increase in muscle cross-section and an improvement in maximal strength.

In our examples of exercise with a partner, the muscular work in most of the exercises is overriding (concentric) as well as elastic (eccentric). Similar exercises can also be carried out without a partner, using either one's own body weight or special equipment (weights, keep-fit devices, rubber tubes).

Why Do Stretching and Strengthening Exercises?

To provide the motivation needed to carry out the exercises presented here, we surely have to answer the question "why?" Even though there is a limited number of scientific publications on the subject of "stretching", the advantages provided by these exercises are well documented. They can be summed up in four key terms:

— Effective flexibility training
— Prevention of sports injuries
— Optimum trainability of the musculature
— Therapeutic benefits in patients with locomotor problems.

Flexibility Training

Static stretching exercises are clearly more effective than the dynamic exercises that include rocking and bouncing (Wallin 1985). Stretching exercises are an essential part of any flexibility training. Flexibility as a condition-determining factor is critical for performance in many sports activities.

A study of competitive skiers has shown that there is marked improvement in flexibility and a decrease in muscular imbalance when stretching exercises are added to the daily exercise program. While practically every athlete was found to have shortened and weakened muscles prior to specific instruction in stretching exercises, far better results were obtained after four years of regular stretching (Spring 1981, 1985, Schmid 1983).

Prevention of Sports Injuries

Muscular imbalance reduces the exercise tolerance of the locomotor system. Shortening and weakening of muscle groups can produce unfavorable loading of joints and, consequently, *overloading of the articular cartilage* (Dietrich 1985). An example is excessive loading at the joint surface behind the patella by a regional muscular imbalance with shortening of the rectus femoris muscle and weakening of the vastus medialis muscle, which plays an extremely important role in the stabilization of the patella.

Tendons of shortened muscles often react with an *inflammation of the tendon attachment* (insertion tendinitis). The principal reason for this is constant overloading of the tendon insertion sites due to shortening of the muscles. Certain muscles have to be optimally stretchable, particularly in sports in which considerable stress is placed on certain tendon attachments by the nature of the activity. A typical example is pain in the groin suffered by soccer players with shortened adductor muscles.

The muscular imbalance interferes with the statics and dynamics of the spine. Shortening of the iliopsoas muscle, the erector spinae muscle, and the rectus femoris muscle, as well as weakening of the abdominal and gluteal muscles, leads to forward tilting of the pelvis and increased lordosis. The resulting reduction in the loading capacity of the spine frequently produces pain and, later, signs of degenerative changes. An effort has to be made to avoid this adverse condition by early initiation of selective stretching and strengthening exercises (Weber 1985).

Shortened, and thus poorly stretchable, muscles are subjected to considerable stress, often exceeding their loading capacity, especially when uncontrolled movements are made. Muscle strains, muscle-fiber tears, and even overt muscle tears result. Conversely, the disturbed relaxation pattern of the shortened muscles can lead to overloading and injury of the contracting antagonist. In the case of a shortened knee extensor, this mechanism may cause injury to the knee flexors (Wyssotschin 1979).

A large-scale study of 12 Swedish soccer teams clearly demonstrated the effectiveness of stretching exercises in preventing sports injuries (Ekstrand 1983).

Optimum Trainability

A shortened tonic muscle can inhibit the maximal activation of its phasic antagonists and synergists. These muscles are consequently weakened. However, strength training to relieve this condition can be fully effective only if the inhibition of the maximal activation is abolished. To accomplish this, the length of the shortened tonic muscle has to be normalized by selective stretching.

Achieving and maintaining muscular balance through regular stretching and strengthening create muscle conditions that permit optimal trainability. This in turn will manifest itself in improved performance.

Therapeutic Use

As soon as a muscular imbalance can be detected, with or without symptoms, stretching and strengthening exercises become effective therapy. In physiotherapy, this method is used in accordance with the individual patient's needs. Long-term success can be achieved only if the patient is motivated to carry out these stretching and strtengthening exercises regularly on his own (Schneider 1984). The desired adaptation of the musculature will come about only by dint of regular training. This exercise therapy has to conform to the relevant training guidelines, which in modified form apply to athletes as well as to patients.

References

Adam K. Modernes Krafttraining im Sport. Berlin: Bartels and Wernitz, 1975.

Akeson WH, Amiel D, Woo S. Immobility effects on synovial joints: the pathomechanics of joint contracture. Biorheology 1980; 17: 95–100.

Alter MJ. Science of stretching. Champaign, IL: Human Kinetics, 1988.

Anderson B. Stretching. Bolinas, CA: Shelter, 1980.

Anderson B. The perfect pre-run stretching routine. Runners World 1978; 13 (5): 56–61.

Asmussen E, Bonde-Petersen F. Storage of elastic energy in skeletal muscles in man. Acta Physiol Scand 1974; 91: 385–92.

Astrand PO, Rodahl K. The textbook of work physiology. 2nd ed. New York: McGraw-Hill, 1974.

Beaulieu JE. Developing a stretching program. Physician Sports Med 1981; 9 (11): 59–69.

Bell RD, Hoshizaki TB. Relationship of age and sex with range of motion of seventeen joint actions in humans. Can J Appl Sports Sci 1981; 6: 202–6.

Blum B, Wöllzenmüller F. Stretching. Bessere Leistungen in allen Sportarten. Oberhaching, West Germany: Sportinform, 1985.

Bryant S. Flexibility and stretching. Physician Sports Med 1984; 12 (2): 171.

Bührle M.: Grundlagen des Maximal- und Schnellkrafttrainings. Schorndorf, West Germany: Hofmann, 1985.

Burkett LN. Investigation into hamstring strains: the case of the hybrid muscle. J Sports Med Phys Fitness 1975; 3: 228–31.

Corbin CB, Noble L. Flexibility: a major component of physical fitness. J Phys Educ Recreation 1980; 51 (6): 23–4, 57–60.

Cornelius WL, Hinson MM. The relationship between isometric contractions of hip extensors and subsequent flexibility in males. J Sports Med Phys Fitness 1980; 20: 75–80.

Crosman LJ, Chateauvert SR, Weisberg J. The effects of massage to the hamstring muscle group on the range of motion. J Orthop Sports Phys Ther 1984; 6: 168–72.

Daniels L, Worthingham C. Muskelfunktionsprüfung. 5th ed. Stuttgart: Fischer, 1985.

Dietrich L, Berthold F, Brenke H. Muskeldehnung aus sportmethodischer Sicht. Med Sport 1985; 25: 52–7.

Ehlenz H, Grosser M, Zimmermann E. Krafttraining. Zurich: BLV, 1983.

Ekstrand J. Gillquist J, Liljedahl SO. Prevention of soccer injuries. Am J Sports Med 1983; 11: 116–20.

Ekstrand J, Gillquist J, Möller M, Oeberg B, Liljedahl SO. Incidence of soccer injuries and their relation to training and team success. Am J Sports Med 1983; 11: 63–7.

Francis KT. Delayed muscle soreness: a review. J Orthop Sports Phys Ther 1983; 5: 10–13.

Harris FA. Facilitation techniques in therapeutic exercise. In: Basmajian JV, ed. Therapeutic exercise. 3rd ed. Baltimore: Williams and Wilkins, 1978: 93–137.

Hettinger T. Isometrisches Muskeltraining. Stuttgart: Thieme, 1983.

Howald H. Morphologische und funktionelle Veränderungen der Muskelfasern durch Training. Schweiz Z Sportmed 1984; 31: 5–14.

Janda V. Muskelfunktionsdiagnostik. Heidelberg: VFM, 1979.

Kahle W, Leonhardt H, Platzer W. Taschenatlas der Anatomie, vol 1. 2nd ed. Stuttgart: Thieme, 1978.

Kapandji IA. The physiology of the joints, vol 1: upper limb. 5th ed. Edinburgh: Churchill Livingstone, 1988.

Kapandji IA. The physiology of the joints, vol 2: lower limb. 5th ed. Edinburgh: Churchill Livingstone, 1988.

Kapandji IA. The physiology of the joints, vol 3: the trunk and vertebral column. 2nd ed. Edinburgh: Churchill Livingstone, 1974.

Kendall HO, Kendall FP, Wadsworth G. Muscle testing and function. 2nd ed. Baltimore: Williams and Wilkins, 1971.

Knebel KP. Funktionsgymnastik. Reinbek, West Germany: Rowohlt, 1985.

Kunz HR, Unold, E. Zielgerichtetes Krafttraining. Trainerinformation (Magglingen) 1986; 20.

Mayhew TP, Norton BJ, Sahrmann SA. Electromyographic study of the relationships between hamstring and abdominal muscles during a unilateral straight leg raise. Phys Ther 1983; 63: 1769–73.

Mellerowicz H, Meller W. Training. 4th ed. Berlin: Springer, 1980.

Moore JC. The Golgi tendon organ: a review and update. Am J Occup Ther 1984; 38: 227–36.

Moore MA, Hutton RS. Electromyographic investigation of muscle stretching techniques. Med Sci Sports 1980; 12: 322–9.

Möller M, Oeberg B, Ekstrand J, Gillquist J. The effect of a strength training program on flexibility [abstract]. Are: Swedish Society of Sports Medicine, 1981.

Newham DJ, Mills KR, Quigley BM, Edwards RHT. Pain and fatigue after concentric and eccentric muscle contractions.

Schmid H, Spring H. Muscular imbalance in skiers. Manual Med 1983; 21: 63–6.

Schmidt RF, Grundriß der Neurophysiologie. 4th ed. Berlin: Springer, 1979.

Schneider, W. Stretching and isometrics. Basle: Roche, 1984.

Schneider W, Dvořák J, Dvořák V, Tritschler T. Manuelle Medizin. Therapie. 2nd ed. Stuttgart: Thieme, 1989.

Schulz H. Stretching: Niedernhausen, West Germany: Falken, 1983.

Shephard RJ. Physiology and biochemistry of exercise. New York: Praeger, 1982.

Smith JL, Hutton RS, Eldred E. Postcontraction changes in sensitivity of muscle afferents to static and dynamic stretch. Brain Res 1974; 78: 193–202.

Sölveborn SA. Das Buch vom Stretching. Munich: Mosaik , 1983.

Spring H. Muskelfunktionsdiagnostik nach Janda. Ergebnisse einer Untersuchung an Skirennfahrern. Schweiz Z Sportmed 1981; 29: 143–6.

Spring H. Was bringt das Stretching? Schweiz Z Sportmed 1985; 33: 21–4.

Stegeman J. Leistungsphysiologie. 3rd ed. Stuttgart: Thieme, 1984.

Stamford B. Flexibility and stretching. Phys Sports Med 1984; 12: 171.

Surburg PR. Neuromuscular facilitation techniques in sports medicine. Phys Sports Med 1981; 18: 114–27.

Travell JG, Simons DG, Myofascial pain and dysfunction: the trigger point manual. Baltimore: Williams and Wilkins, 1983.

Vries HA de. Physical fitness programs: does physical activity promote relaxation? J Phys Educ Recreation 1975; 46 (7): 52–3.

Tittel K. Beschreibende und funktionelle Anatomie des Menschen. 9th ed. Stuttgart: Fischer, 1981.

Uram P. The complete stretching book. Mountain View, CA: Anderson World, 1980.

Wallin D., Ekblom B, Grahn R, Nordenborg T. Improvement of muscle flexibility: a comparison between two techniques. Am J Sports Med 1985; 13: 263–8.

Weber J, Berthold F, Brenke H, Dietrich L. Die Bedeutung muskulärer Dysbalancen für die Störung der arthromuskulären Beziehungen. Med Sport 1985; 25: 149–51.

Weineck J. Optimales Training. Erlangen, West Germany: Perimed, 1980.

Weineck J. Sportanatomie. 3rd ed. Erlangen, West Germany: Perimed, 1983.

Wiktorssohn-Möller M, Öberg B, Ekstrand J, Gillquist J. Effects of warming up, massage, and stretching on range of motion and muscle strength in the lower extremity. Am J Sports Med 1983; 11: 249–52.

Wilmore J, Parr RB, Girandola RN, et al. Physiological alterations consequent to circuit weight training. Med Sci Sport 1978; 10: 79–84.

Williams JCP, Sperryn PN. Sports medicine. 2nd ed. Baltimore: Williams and Wilkins, 1976.

Wolff HD. Neurophysiologische Aspekte der manuellen Medizin. 2nd ed. Berlin: Springer, 1983.

Wyssotschin IW. Die Polymyographie. Eine Methode zur Untersuchung des Funktionszustandes des neuromuskulären Systems bei Sportlern. Med Sport 1979; 19: 361–4.